615.892
B777a

DETROIT PUBLIC LIBRARY

28 1

D0060803

Acupuncture:
efficacy, safety and practice

BST

Acupuncture:
efficacy, safety and practice

Board of Science and Education
British Medical Association

harwood academic publishers

Australia • Canada • France • Germany • India • Japan
Luxembourg • Malaysia • The Netherlands • Russia
Singapore • Switzerland • Thailand • United Kingdom

615.892
B 277 a

OCT 12 '01

Copyright © 2000 British Medical Association
Published by license under the Harwood Academic Publishers imprint,
part of The Gordon and Breach Publishing Group.

All rights reserved.

No part of this book may be reproduced or utilized in any form or by
any means, electronic or mechanical, including photocopying and
recording, or by any information storage or retrieval system, without
permission in writing from the publisher. Printed in the United
Kingdom.

Amsteldijk 166
1st Floor
1079 LH Amsterdam
The Netherlands

British Library Cataloguing in Publication Data

A catalogue record for this book is available from the British Library.

ISBN 90-5823-164-X (soft cover)

Cover photograph: Telegraph Colour Library

Ts

BETROIT PUBLIC LIBRARY
TECHNOLOGY & SCIENCE

Contents

Editorial Board

A publication from the BMA Science Department and the Board of Science and Education.

Chairman, Board of Science and Education	Sir William Asscher
Head of Professional Resources and Research Group	Professor Vivienne Nathanson
Editor	Dr David Morgan
Research and writing	Laura Conway
Contributors	Marcia Darvell
	Lisa Davies
	Professor Edzard Ernst
	Hilary Forrester
	Kate Thomas
	Dr Adrian White
Editorial secretariat	Nicholas Harrison
	Dawn Whyndham
Indexer	Richard Jones

Board of Science and Education

This report was prepared under the auspices of the Board of Science and Education of the British Medical Association, whose membership for 1999/00 was as follows:

Sir Peter Froggatt	President, BMA
Professor B R Hopkinson	Chairman, Representative Body, BMA
Dr I G Bogle	Chairman of BMA Council
Dr W J Appleyard	Treasurer, BMA
Sir William Asscher	Chairman, Board of Science and Education
Dr P H Dangerfield	Deputy Chairman, Board of Science and Education

Dr A Elsharkawy
Dr H W K Fell
Dr R Gupta (Deputy)
Dr S Hajioff
Dr V Leach
Dr N D L Olsen
Professor M R Rees
Dr S J Richards
Miss S Somjee
Dr P Steadman (Deputy)
Dr S Taylor
Dr D M B Ward

Approval for publication as a BMA policy report was recommended by BMA Executive Committee of Council on 7th June 2000.

Acknowledgements

The Association is grateful for the help provided by the BMA Committees and many outside experts and organisations, and would particularly like to thank: Dr Joel Bonnet, Dr Imogen Evans, Val Hopwood, Simon Fielding, Simon Mills, Felicity Moir, the acupuncture organisations listed in Appendix II, Butterworth-Heinemann, and the researchers who provided information about their current work. We are also indebted to the GP members who took time to provide us with detailed responses to our postal survey.

List of tables

List of figures

1
Introduction

The British Medical Association (BMA) Board of Science and Education was established to support the Association in its founding aim 'to promote the medical and allied sciences and to maintain the honour and interests of the medical profession'. Part of the remit of the Board is to undertake research studies on a wide range of key public health issues on behalf of the Association and to provide reports and guidance to the profession and information to the public on health related matters which are of general concern. When endorsed by BMA Council, the reports are published as BMA policy reports to influence doctors, Government, policy makers, the professions, the media and the public. Over the past two decades particularly, the Board has helped to formulate BMA policy on complementary and alternative medicine (CAM) and published two major reports (BMA, 1986; BMA, 1993).

Growth in the use of Complementary and Alternative Medicine (CAM)

The NHS spends considerable money on the treatment of chronic and undifferentiated disease, conditions for which patients often seek help from CAM. The Office of Health Economics in 1991 recorded an NHS expenditure of £1 billion per annum with respect to these conditions, which in 2000 is likely to be exceeded. By 1995 it was estimated that 39.5% of GP partnerships in England were providing access to complementary therapy for their NHS patients (Thomas *et al.*, 1995).

This provision may be via the primary care team itself, referral to one of six NHS homoeopathic hospitals, to pain clinics or to private practitioners, or through the employment of complementary practitioners in GP practices. Thomas *et al.* (2000) estimated that the NHS provided 10% of contacts to six established CAM therapies (acupuncture, medical herbalism, chiropractic, osteopathy, homoeopathy and hypnotherapy) in the year 1997/8.

In its second report to the Department of Health, the Centre for Complementary Health Studies in Exeter estimated that up to 5 million people may have consulted a practitioner specialising in CAM in the last year, and an incalculable extra number may have consulted a statutory health professional practising CAM (Mills and Budd, 2000). Up to one third of UK cancer patients use complementary therapies and many oncology units and hospices offer at least one CAM therapy to patients (Kohn, 1999). Acupuncture and homoeopathy are the most commonly provided therapies, and acupuncture is now reported to be available in 86% of NHS chronic pain services (DoH, 1999).

Current estimates indicate that there could be more than 60,000 CAM practitioners and possibly 20,000 statutory health professionals regularly practising a variety of CAM therapies in the UK. Of these, there are about 2,050 acupuncture practitioners (an increase of 36% in two years) and 3,530 statutory health practitioners practising acupuncture (an increase of 51% in two years).

The rapid growth in popularity of CAM suggests a greater degree of public awareness with what they may see as the limitations of orthodox medicine and concern over the side effects of ever more potent drugs (FIM, 1997). It coincides with the growing view within conventional healthcare practice that a renewed emphasis needs to be placed on the patient-doctor relationship and on seeing patients as individuals in the personal and social settings in which their problems develop. This view is reflected in both the GMC's 1993 report, *Tomorrow's Doctors,* and the BMA's report, *Complementary Medicine: New Approaches to Good Practice,* published in the same year. It is also consistent with the current emphasis in the NHS of basing treatment on proven effectiveness and on value for money.

A shift in attitude within the medical profession is reflected in the BMA's present policy and in the use of the term 'complementary' rather than 'alternative'. A large national postal survey of GPs showed that many have an 'open mind' as to the value of such treatments (GMSC, 1992), with many GP partnerships in England providing access to some form of complementary therapy for NHS patients (Thomas *et al.*, 1995).

Writing in 1998, the President of the Royal College of Physicians of London (RCP) commented, "we can no longer ignore the existence of alternative therapies ... we, in the Royal College of Physicians, have established a committee to advise the college on how we should handle the alternative therapies. Disbelief among conventional practitioners has at least been replaced by a healthy skepticism and a clear wish to examine the evidence sensibly and logically" (RCP, 1998). The RCP has since sent a questionnaire to its members to gauge their use of CAM and attitude towards it.

BMA policy on CAM

The 1993 BMA policy report continues to reflect the Association's policy on CAM. Patients are increasingly asking doctors about CAM therapies, and it is currently difficult for patients and doctors to identify those therapists who are competent and adequately trained to carry out such treatments. Doctors are duty bound to delegate care only to those whom they believe are competent, and it may be important for the patient's doctor to maintain continuing clinical control of the patient's treatment. While medical practitioners are free to practise whatever form of medicine is appropriate for the patient, they remain accountable to the General Medical Council for all treatments. However, how can doctors be certain that their patients are safe when delivered into the hands of a CAM practitioner?

The BMA's policies on CAM have reflected a particular interest in the *discrete clinical disciplines* of homoeopathy, osteopathy, chiropractic, acupuncture and herbal medicine. These are distinguished from other therapies by having more established foundations of training, are increasingly the therapies of choice for the UK public, but also have in common the greatest potential to do harm to the patient directly, since they involve physical manipulation or invasive techniques, and/or by misdiagnosis or omission (BMA, 1993).

Last year the BMA's General Practitioner Committee (GPC) issued guidance on referrals to complementary therapists indicating that GPs can safely *refer* patients to complementary therapists who are registered as doctors or nurses, and also to registered practitioners in osteopathy and chiropractic, and confirmed that GPs can *delegate* treatment to other CAM practitioners, subject to a number of criteria (GPC, 1999). In delegating to a CAM practitioner GPs are advised to:

- Satisfy themselves that the treatment seems appropriate and is likely to benefit the patient

- Pass on any necessary information about the patient to the therapist, with the patient's clear consent

- Retain responsibility for managing the patient's care (as stated by the GMC, 1998).

Annual Representative Meeting 1998 policy

The 1998 BMA Annual Representative Meeting raised issues concerning efficacy and safety, with specific reference to acupuncture, and the following resolution was passed:

"That this Representative Body asks the Board of Science [and Education] to investigate the scientific basis and efficacy of acupuncture and the quality of training and standards of competence in its practitioners".

The BMA Board of Science and Education has undertaken a comprehensive review of some of the major aspects of acupuncture, examining the published literature, obtaining education and training information from acupuncture organisations, universities and so forth, and communicating with practitioners. Importantly, a national postal survey of a random sample of GPs was undertaken in 1999 which has provided new comprehensive data and information about GPs' knowledge and use of acupuncture in the UK today.

To ensure that a wide range of views was obtained in support of this study, the BMA science secretariat sought information from the main organisations which act as professional bodies for acupuncturists from the comprehensive list provided by the University of Exeter (Mills and Peacock, 1997; Mills and Budd, 2000) (see Appendix II).

Scope of the report

The majority of issues considered in this report, such as safety, efficacy and training, are important to all users of acupuncture, whether NHS patients, or private, self-referred patients. However, the issue of cost-effectiveness applies most strongly to its provision in the NHS, and not to private practices. With 90% of the consultations being private, an estimated £450 million per annum is spent on out-of-pocket fees for treatment (Thomas *et al.*, 2000).

This first chapter has provided background to the BMA's policies on CAM and the remit of this report. The question of the clinical effectiveness and efficacy of acupuncture treatment for a variety of medical conditions is addressed in chapter 2, where the results of key clinical trials are summarised. Chapters 3 and 4 discuss the important issues of the safety of acupuncture, and the training and education of its practitioners. The main results of the BMA 1999 postal survey of UK GPs are presented in chapter 5, gauging the attitudes and knowledge that GPs have about acupuncture, and the extent to which it is being offered to patients. Finally, future developments in the provision of CAM, particularly acupuncture, are examined in chapter 6, including funding and research issues, cost-effectiveness, and its integration into the NHS. The BMA's recommendations for future action are presented.

2
The evidence base of acupuncture

Introduction

The study and practice of complementary and alternative medicine (CAM) is now at a new crossroads. In the West, the growth in the number and variety of CAM therapies is a fairly recent phenomenon, and the rate of patient consultations for treatments is increasing rapidly (Eisenberg *et al.*, 1998), with 'snapshots' in time illustrating this phenomenon (Eisenberg *et al.*, 1993; Thomas *et al.*, 1995; MacLennan *et al.*, 1996; Ernst and White, 2000). With this increase comes the question of its position within the UK healthcare system, and whether the time has come to aim for its integration into the NHS. For this to occur, a sound evidence base of the therapies' efficacy is required.

Practitioners of acupuncture generally follow one of two broad theoretical bases, Traditional Chinese Medicine (TCM) or Western acupuncture. Acupuncture research is complicated by the number and diversity of practices and schools of instruction (see chapter 4). Each may use a different approach and most are based on the concepts of TCM, although there is a growing interest in purely biomedical or Western acupuncture. Since there is no evidence that any one approach is superior, this report does not distinguish between the training or techniques covered by individual schools or courses.

Traditional Chinese Medicine

Complementary medicine and 'natural therapies' have their origins in the civilisations of Babylon, Egypt and China, of about 3,000 years ago. The Chinese developed a system of medicine based on an extraordinarily detailed knowledge of herbal remedies, combined with acupuncture. TCM is practised through an holistic approach and focuses on the unity of the human body with its environment.

The TCM picture of the human body presents a construction of 'energetic functions', as opposed to the traditional Western view of the body based on structure (anatomy) and function (physiology), with the various parts operating together as systems in a mechanical manner. TCM suggests that about 365 acupuncture points are present on the human body, arranged in lines or channels (meridians) — there are 12 main meridians along which energy or 'Qi' flows in a coherent and ordered manner. If the flow is interrupted for any reason, then ill health can occur. It is thought by some that acupuncture is preventive medicine, enabling them to maintain and improve their level of health, perhaps even enhancing an individual's resistance to infections. In illness, acupuncture seeks to stimulate the appropriate 'point' along the affected channel, permitting the energy to become balanced and to flow freely once more. Diagnosis is based on close examination of the patient's tongue and pulse, with careful questioning to explore the signs and symptoms of the diseases. Treatments are based on the evaluation of the diagnosis to rebalance the Yin and Yang deficiency or excess in the body (ie, the negative and positive polarisations of Qi).

The 'Western' approach to acupuncture

The 'Western' approach to acupuncture, as often practised in the UK, is a non-traditional version based on modern concepts of neuroanatomy and physiology. This considers the 'gate theory' of pain, acting via the nervous, endocrine and immune systems, rather than the traditional theory of meridians. Fewer needles may be used and are left *in situ* for a much shorter time compared to TCM practice. An important concept is that of the 'trigger point' – an area of increased sensitivity within a muscle thought to cause a characteristic pattern of referred pain in a related area of the body.

This brief report cannot explore the theories and practice that make up the art and science of acupuncture in detail. Readers are advised to consult specialist literature; two new contributions from Harwood Academic Publishers are currently 'in press' (Chan and Lee, in press; Cheung, Li and Wong, in press). However the chapters that follow are based on a comprehensive study of the published literature from peer-reviewed journals and present an up-to-date review of the efficacy, safety and application of acupuncture in the UK.

Views on acupuncture

Practitioners of some CAM therapies support the view that science does have a place within their fields of practice. Concepts of 'science-based', 'evidence-based' and 'placebo-controlled' are being discussed, with new research trials planned or underway.

Some major providers of complementary medicine within the NHS, such as the Royal London Homoeopathic Hospital (RLHH), are clearly seeking to establish CAM as a form of evidence-based medicine. This CAM centre provides a range of different CAM treatments including acupuncture, and has an ongoing programme of research involving clinical trials, clinical audit and literature reviews. These have concluded that there is "strong evidence that acupuncture can have specific therapeutic effects" (RLHH, 1999).

For others, traditional concepts of life force, Qi, energy, potentisation, and 'healing' continue to be of greater importance than the science base of the therapies. The holistic approach aims to treat the whole person, and may lead to an improvement in the patient by inducing a feeling of wellbeing, even if the physical condition is not markedly improved. However, this does not preclude the measurement of outcomes, and it is necessary to identify the appropriate ones. The relationship between the therapist and patient, the degree of confidence inspired within the patient for both therapy and therapist, and any placebo effect, could be significant factors in achieving a successful outcome.

A number of differing views on the value of acupuncture have been expressed by key organisations. The World Health Organization encourages and supports countries to identify safe and effective remedies and practices for acupuncture use in public and private health services, and has produced guidelines on basic training and safety in acupuncture (WHO, 1999). The Royal Society, in providing evidence to the House of Lords Inquiry (1999) on CAM, reported that meta-analyses of published studies have largely shown "beneficial effects for the treatment of pain" but commented that reports may show publication bias (i.e. the selective publication of papers).

However, the European Commission in their five-year study ("Co-operation in Science and Technology Action B4", 1998) of unconventional medicine, concluded that the only good evidence available for the effectiveness of acupuncture was for nausea and vomiting, while the evidence for the effectiveness of acupuncture in the treatment of various painful conditions, smoking cessation and asthma, was not convincing. Despite this, they conclude, "acupuncture...is recommended by a number of experts and organisations including the World Health Organization". The American National Institutes of Health concluded in their consensus statement (1997) that promising results have emerged, for example in adult postoperative and chemotherapy nausea and vomiting, and in postoperative dental pain. They stated, "there is sufficient evidence of acupuncture's value to expand its use into conventional medicine and to encourage further studies of its physiology and clinical value".

Ernst and White (1999a) have recently published a comprehensive appraisal of acupuncture, commenting, "since the development of the concept of evidence-based healthcare, therapies must establish their efficacy, safety and cost-effectiveness by means of rigorous studies". Indeed they suggest that scientific validation of CAM therapies has become an ethical imperative due to its prevalence in the UK (Ernst and White, 2000). Information on the evidence base of acupuncture should help doctors, patients, researchers and purchasers of healthcare become more informed on the value of acupuncture and its likely place within the NHS.

Clinical trials of acupuncture

In conventional medicine the randomised controlled trial (RCT) is the 'gold standard' of evidence (van Haselen and Fisher, 1999), hence there is a call for the same standard to be used for unconventional medicine. In a RCT, patients for whom a certain treatment may be of benefit are randomly allocated to a treatment or control group and followed forward in time. If participants are unaware of their assigned status, then they are said to be 'blinded' or 'masked'. Studies where only the research participants are unaware of their assigned status are known as 'single-blind' studies, whereas when both the research participants and the investigators are unaware of their assigned status, the studies are known as 'double-blind'.

Trials of acupuncture must be 'single blind', as the acupuncturist is aware if the participant is in the control group where a placebo is being administered (Filshie and White, 1998). Different forms of control procedures have emerged: sham acupuncture can be employed, involving needling away from classical point locations. Sham acupuncture has been shown to have some clinical effect mainly due to placebo, although this is most marked in painful conditions and nausea (Filshie and White, 1998). However, it has been difficult to find suitable sham acupuncture techniques that appear indistinguishable from a needle, yet are inert. Tapping the skin, placing needles only superficially, or needling the wrong points, have been used, but are likely to produce a physiological response similar to needling and thus lead to an underestimate of the effect of acupuncture. This problem appears to have been solved recently (Streitberger and Kleinhenz, 1998) with the development of a placebo acupuncture needle which appears to result in a similar sensation to a normal acupuncture needle without actually piercing the skin.

Randomised controlled trials can provide evidence of whether acupuncture can work, but only in an experimental setting on a selected group of patients. A further form of clinical trial is known as the pragmatic randomised controlled trial, where studies using random allocation to intervention or control groups are used to compare two different treatments. They are designed to assess the comparative effectiveness of the different treatments as they are delivered in a real world setting. In the context of acupuncture research, their aim would be to determine whether it is better than other available treatment options. Cost-effectiveness assessments can also be made using this methodology. Cost-effectiveness is a comparative concept – treatment can only be more or less cost-effective than some other form of management or treatment (Thomas and Fitter, 1997).

This chapter evaluates the evidence for and against the effectiveness of acupuncture, based on systematic reviews of controlled clinical trials for the following conditions:

• Back pain (Ernst and White, 1998)

• Neck pain (White and Ernst, 1999)

• Osteoarthritis (Ernst, 1997a)

• Recurrent headache (Melchart *et al.*, 1999)

• Nausea and vomiting (Vickers, 1996)

• Smoking cessation (White *et al.*, 1999)

• Weight loss (Ernst, 1997b)

• Stroke (Ernst and White, 1996)

• Dental pain (Ernst and Pittler, 1998)

A thorough search of all published controlled clinical trials on each subject was conducted by the researchers listed above, with precedence being given to trials in which the design controlled for placebo effects. The search strategies used in the majority of these reviews are summarised in table 1 (see page 26). The full details of each review can be found in the respective reports. The papers for each review were chosen according to predefined inclusion/exclusion criteria, followed by standardised data extraction and (where possible) data synthesis.

The majority of RCTs have been conducted according to the Western approach to acupuncture. Acupuncture administered using the TCM philosophy is often accompanied by the use of herbs and a different diagnostic procedure to orthodox medicine (although elements of orthodox diagnosis may be used). High quality research in this area is to be encouraged, both to assess its efficacy for different conditions, and to ensure the safety of the herbs used.

Acupuncture for back pain

A systematic review and meta-analysis of acupuncture for back pain located twelve RCTs (Ernst and White, 1998). Quality was assessed by the Jadad score (Jadad *et al.*, 1996). Several methods for assessing the quality of studies have been devised, but most have the disadvantage that there is no basis for scoring the different items. The Jadad method is derived from research with blinded assessors, and was demonstrated to measure the quality of studies reliably. Points (up to a maximum of five) are awarded for randomisation, blinding and description of withdrawals and drop-outs. In addition to this assessment, the adequacy of the acupuncture for back pain was also assessed by six medical acupuncturists in a blinded study. There was sufficient agreement to separate the trials into three levels of adequacy of acupuncture.

Of the twelve included studies of back pain (see table 2, page 28), nine provided details of responder rate and could be combined in a meta-analysis. A total of 377 participants were included. Six of these studies reached the threshold of three points on the Jadad scale. The overall Odds Ratio was 2.30 (95% CI 1.28-4.13), indicating that acupuncture was significantly better than various control interventions. The results of three out of the twelve studies were markedly more positive, but no explanation for this could be found. Combining the results of the four placebo controlled studies produced an Odds Ratio of 1.37

(95% CI 0.84-2.25), indicating that there was no significant difference between real and placebo acupuncture.

A subsequent review (van Tulder *et al.*, 1999) of essentially the same studies used different assessment criteria, concluding that the studies could not be combined in a meta-analysis since the form of acupuncture used and type of participants involved were not sufficiently homogeneous. They concluded that because the review did not clearly indicate that acupuncture is effective in the management of low back pain, they would not recommend it as a regular treatment for patients with low back pain.

However, as van Tulder and colleagues pointed out themselves, the levels of evidence used in their review were arbitrary, since there is no agreement on how to assess the strength of evidence. Other levels of evidence could lead to different conclusions. The Jadad score was used for quality assessment in Ernst and White's (1998) review, and indeed a different conclusion was reached. In terms of the heterogeneity of the studies, although different forms of acupuncture were used in the studies, it is likely that there was a commonality at least of point-selection: all involved treatment using either classical acupuncture points in the area of the pain, or tender/trigger points in the associated muscles. It would therefore seem reasonable to combine the results of these studies under the general heading of 'acupuncture'. Patient populations were diverse, some having leg pain as well as back pain, and some having previously undergone back surgery. The inclusion of patients with diverse diagnoses should not be particularly problematic since acupuncture treatment would not be altered drastically to account for symptoms, and in any case this diversity would tend to bias the results against acupuncture rather than being in favour. Therefore, the balance of evidence does seem to suggest that acupuncture can be useful in the treatment of back pain.

There is clearly a need for more research into the use of acupuncture for back pain. At present, the NHS is funding a pragmatic randomised controlled trial into the clinical and economic benefits of providing acupuncture services to patients with low back pain assessed as suitable for primary care management (Thomas *et al.*, 1999).

Acupuncture for neck pain

A systematic review found fourteen RCTs which compared acupuncture (White and Ernst, 1999) with various interventions for the treatment of neck pain (see table 3, page 30). Half scored at least three points on the Jadad scale. The overall results of these studies were precisely balanced, with seven positive and seven negative. Looking at the individual comparisons, acupuncture was superior to waiting list (that is, no additional treatment) in one study, and either equal to or superior to physiotherapy in three studies. In five studies, needling did not prove to be superior to placebo controls. The clinical impression exists among acupuncturists that neck pain usually responds well to acupuncture.

This review concludes that neck pain does improve with acupuncture, but there is no clear evidence that this is due to the needling or the overall effect of the therapeutic encounter.

Acupuncture for osteoarthritis

Thirteen studies were identified in a systematic review of acupuncture for osteoarthritis in any joint, (Ernst, 1997) of which seven reported a positive result and six a negative one (see table 4, page 32). Of the positive studies, the majority failed to control for placebo effects. Of the five placebo-controlled studies, four found no difference between the effect of acupuncture and the effect of sham. As with neck pain, it is unclear whether the clinical benefits which many patients experience from acupuncture are a specific or a non-specific response.

Acupuncture for recurrent headache

In a systematic review of RCTs for migraine and tension headache, 22 RCTs were included (see table 5, page 33) (Melchart *et al.*, 1999). The quality of studies was variable, with a median Jadad score of two. Acupuncture was compared to sham acupuncture in 14 studies, the majority of which showed at least a trend in favour of acupuncture. Pooled results for the responder ratios were 1.55 (95% CI 1.04-2.33) for migraine and 1.49 (95% CI 0.96-2.30) for tension headache. The authors concluded that, overall, the existing evidence suggests that acupuncture has a role in the treatment of recurrent headache but the quality and amount of evidence is not fully convincing.

Nausea and vomiting

For the treatment of nausea and vomiting, acupuncture is usually given at a single site, known as P6 on the inner wrist. An early review found 33 controlled trials of acupuncture (and related forms of stimulation) for nausea and vomiting either postoperatively, or in early pregnancy or due to chemotherapy (see table 5, page 33) (Vickers, 1996). In four trials, the acupuncture was given under anaesthetic: all these were negative. Of the remaining 29 trials, 27 demonstrated a significant effect of acupuncture compared to various control procedures.

In a subsequent review restricted to treatment for nausea in pregnancy (Murphy, 1998), seven studies on acupressure were found, but none on acupuncture. (Acupressure involves the stimulation of acupuncture points by finger pressure rather then needles). The reliability of the studies and success of the control interventions were called into question, and an additional rigorous study was included, which had a negative outcome. Murphy concluded that acupuncture seemed to be both safe and probably helpful to pregnant women with nausea, but that it was far from clear whether this effect depended on the precise positioning of the stimulus.

A meta-analysis of acupuncture for postoperative nausea and vomiting (Lee and Done, 1999) combined 19 studies involving 1,679 participants. The median Jadad score was three. In four studies involving children, there were no differences between P6 stimulation and control groups for nausea or vomiting at any time period. In adults, the results favoured P6 stimulation over sham controls for both nausea experienced within six hours after surgery (relative risk 0.34, 95% CI 0.20-0.58) and vomiting experienced within six hours after surgery (relative risk 0.47, 95% CI 0.34-0.64). Numbers needed to treat, that is, the number of patients that would need to receive acupuncture to avoid nausea or vomiting in one patient compared with the control condition, were four (3 to 6) and five (4 to 8) respectively. Sample size or types of control did not affect this result, but when the analysis for nausea was restricted to high quality studies the result was no longer significant. The results for nausea and vomiting experienced 0-48 hours after surgery did not find that P6 stimulation was superior to placebo. The results also show that P6 stimulation has equivalent effectiveness to antiemetic drugs in preventing vomiting, both shortly after surgery (0-6 hours), and a while after surgery (up to 48 hours after).

Stimulation of the P6 point has also been implicated in the prevention of motion sickness (Gahlinger, 1999), and wristbands can be purchased as a therapeutic aid. One study of such bands found no evidence of a reduction in motion sickness symptoms (Bruce *et al.*, 1990), but a possible reason for this failure was the infrequent stimulation of the point due to lack of wrist movement. In a later study, however, which

DETROIT PUBLIC LIBRARY
TECHNOLOGY & SCIENCE

involved regular manual pulse pressure of the P6 point, a significant reduction in the severity of symptoms was found (Hu *et al.*, 1995).

Acupuncture for smoking cessation and weight loss

Acupuncture has gained a reputation for assisting the management of certain behaviours, particularly smoking (see table 6, page 34) and over-eating. A Cochrane Review for smoking (White *et al.*, 1999) included 18 reports with 20 trials which compared acupuncture to various control interventions. Acupuncture was no better than placebo acupuncture, whether assessed immediately after treatment or at six or twelve-month follow-ups. On the basis of three studies, acupuncture was better than no treatment at all immediately, but this benefit had disappeared by six months.

A systematic review of acupuncture for weight loss found four studies (Ernst, 1997). Their quality was poor: the two most rigorous studies were negative and the two less rigorous were positive. Thus, at present there is no evidence to support any role for acupuncture in the management of smoking cessation or weight loss.

Acupuncture for stroke

Six controlled trials of acupuncture treatment to assist recovery from stroke were reviewed (see table 7, page 34) (Ernst and White, 1996). All showed some benefit of acupuncture compared to the control intervention. None of these trials was placebo-controlled, so it is impossible to say whether the effect was due to the placement and stimulation of the needles, or due to the extra attention and mental stimulation given to the subjects. In a more recent study, (Gosman-Hedstroem *et al.*, 1998) this question seems to have been answered in acupuncture's disfavour. This rigorous, placebo-controlled RCT found no effect of either genuine or placebo acupuncture compared to a group who had no additional treatment. The interaction between acupuncturists and patients was strictly controlled and minimised. Collectively, these data suggest that the effects of acupuncture in improving the recovery from stroke are mostly non-specific in nature.

Acupuncture for dental pain

Dental pain provides an accessible, temporary and relatively reproducible model for testing the analgesic effect of acupuncture. It has been studied both in laboratory experiments and during actual dental surgery; 16 controlled trials of either sort of dental pain were included in a systematic review (see table 8, page 36). The quality of the studies was generally poor, with only two scoring at least three out of a possible five points on the Jadad scale. The great majority of studies suggest that acupuncture does have an effect greater than placebo in reducing dental pain. In particular, all four studies of acupuncture for experimental dental pain were positive. Of the eight studies in which some blinding was incorporated, only one was negative. This suggests that acupuncture does have genuine effects in reducing dental pain, though the effect is small and probably not important clinically. This result has theoretical importance in indicating that acupuncture can have measurable analgesic effects.

Other conditions

Systematic reviews of acupuncture for fibromyalgia, (Berman *et al.*, 1999) and temporomandibular joint dysfunction (Ernst and White, 1999b) have promising results but more research is required, particularly sham-controlled RCTs. Systematic reviews of acupuncture for asthma (Linde *et al.*, 2000), rheumatic diseases (Lautenschlaeger, 1997), and for tinnitus (Park, *et al.* in press) have shown no evidence of an effect in these conditions.

Summary

According to the current evidence, acupuncture appears to be more effective than sham acupuncture or other control interventions for nausea and vomiting (most convincing for post-operative symptoms in adults), and for back pain, dental pain and migraine. The present evidence is unclear as to whether the response of osteoarthritis and neck pain to acupuncture is more than non-specific. Acupuncture's role in recovery from stroke, and the treatment of tension headache, fibromyalgia and temporomandibular joint dysfunction is still uncertain. Acupuncture appears not to be superior to sham acupuncture for smoking cessation or weight loss.

Methodological difficulties

Research in complementary and alternative medicine in general is limited by lack of funding, lack of research skills, lack of an academic infrastructure and lack of patients (RLHH, 1999). In 1996 only 0.08% of research funding in the NHS was allocated to complementary medicine (Ernst, 1996). In addition, clinical trials are not without their critics; they have been criticised for investigating conditions and using treatment techniques which may not be representative of those treated and used in practice (RLHH, 1999). The use of the randomised controlled trial in acupuncture studies has been considered a particular intellectual challenge, as it is often considered that there are more potential difficulties than in the randomised, double-blind, crossover controlled clinical trials used to evaluate pharmaceutical agents.

A common assertion among skeptics is that the results of complementary therapies, including acupuncture, are built solely on what is known as the placebo effect, that is, an improvement in the condition of an ill individual that occurs in response to treatment but cannot be considered due to the specific treatment used. The placebo effect is often considered in a pejorative sense, as it is confused with the 'non-specific noise' of placebo that must be eliminated from clinical trials in order to determine the effectiveness of particular pharmacological interventions (Harrington, 1997). However, the placebo effect may have a value for patients. Cochrane, an early advocate of the randomised controlled trial and former director of the Medical Research Council's Epidemiology Unit, indicated that 'effectiveness' due to placebo should not be discounted without consideration of the economic effects. He argued (Black *et al.*, 1984) that the use of placebos in the correct place should be encouraged, but that what is inefficient, is the use of relatively expensive drugs as placebos. Further research is required to investigate the presence of a placebo effect in acupuncture, comparing acupuncture with sham acupuncture and other placebo controls.

Clearly, in real clinical situations, effectiveness and efficacy include issues such as cost-effectiveness and clinical safety, as well as issues related to clinical trials. The placebo effect in itself should not be a reason for discounting complementary therapy research, as the usefulness of a medical intervention in practice is different from assessing formal efficacy (NIH, 1997). It has been stated that one possible advantage for acupuncture use is that the incidence of adverse effects is "substantially lower than that of many drugs or other accepted medical procedures used for the same condition." (NIH, 1997). In a recent survey of GPs and directors of public health in the UK (van Haselen and Fisher, 1999) it was found that although randomised controlled trials and safety were the key considerations for the purchasing of complementary therapies, "audit outcome data from homoeopathic hospitals, economic evaluation and availability of literature" were also rated highly for importance. The European Committee for Homoeopathy also recently emphasised the importance of effectiveness research – for example, using observational studies (European Committee for Homeopathy 1997), and Black (1996) called for the advocates of RCTs and the advocates of observational studies to work in mutual recognition of the complementary roles of the two approaches.

However, the randomised controlled clinical trial, and the pragmatic RCT, remain important linchpins of medical research. Although they may be considered in conjunction with other forms of research such as observational techniques, acupuncture research must provide evidence of clinical efficacy which enables acupuncture techniques to be compared with conventional medicine.

Future research

The Royal London Homoeopathic Hospital (1999) has identified questions that need to be answered by research in the field of complementary medicine, which can be applied specifically to acupuncture research:

• How large is the effect of acupuncture?

• Are the overall long-term effects of a acupuncture treatment greater than some reasonable alternative such as surgery or drug treatment?

• How cost-effective is acupuncture?

• Is acupuncture additional to, or can it replace, conventional treatments such as drugs?

• Which conditions is acupuncture most effective for?

• Which patients benefit most from acupuncture?

Randomised controlled trials with rigorous methodological controls are essential if medical practitioners are to make decisions for referral to acupuncturists based on a scientific basis. However, it may also be the case that '*complementary research*' is required in order to answer some of the questions above and provide a full picture of the effectiveness and efficacy of acupuncture in clinical practice – for example, case studies, health status measurement (Jenkinson and McGee, 1998), cost-effectiveness analysis and observational studies (Black, 1996). Such a combination of research methods, including the randomised controlled trial, may provide answers to the outstanding questions raised by the Royal London Homoeopathic

Hospital, but it is clear that current standards of research into the clinical effectiveness of acupuncture require greater methodological rigour.

Finally, it is important to consider that effectiveness measures in clinical trials do not take into consideration the comparative merits of particular forms of treatment. As health service resources are finite, considerations of cost and unwanted effects of particular treatments need to be considered. In the UK, the National Institute of Clinical Excellence has been established to consider the value of particular treatments in clinical practice, and is well placed to consider acupuncture and produce guidance for the NHS.

Table 1: Summary of methodological details of reviews of the clinical effectiveness of acupuncture

Project/reference	Acupuncture type	Databases searched
Dental pain (Ernst and Pittler, 1998)	Any	Medline, Embase, CISCOM Cochrane library, Own files
Low back pain (Ernst and White, 1998)	Needle only, with or without electrical stimulation	Medline, CISCOM Cochrane library, Own files
Neck pain (White and Ernst, 1999)	Any	Medline, Embase, Cochrane library CISCOM, Own files
Osteoarthritis (Ernst, 1997a)	Any	Medline, CISCOM, Own files
Stroke (Ernst and White, 1996)	Any	Medline, CISCOM, Own files
Smoking cessation (White et al, in press)	Any	Medline, Embase, British Library, CISCOM, Science Citation Index, Own files
Weight loss (Ernst, 1997b)	Any acup or acupressure	Medline, CISCOM, Own files

Main inclusion criteria	Main exclusion criteria
Controlled trials on human volunteers/patients	Trials comparing one form of acup vs another
RCTs on human patients	Trials comparing one form of acup vs another
	Trials published in languages other than English,
	French, German, Spanish, Italian or Polish
RCTs	Headache only or pain in multiple sites
	Trials comparing one form of acup vs another
Controlled trials on human patients	Trials comparing one form of acup vs another
Controlled trials on human patients	Trials comparing one form of acup vs another
Sham-controlled, single-blind	Trials published in languages other than English,
RCTs on smokers	French or German
Randomised, sham-controlled trials	Trials comparing one form of acup vs another

Source: Ernst E (1999). Clinical effectiveness of acupuncture: an overview of systematic reviews. In E Ernst & A White (eds.) Acupuncture: a scientific appraisal. Oxford: Butterworth-Heinemann Reprinted by permission of Butterworth-Heinemann

Table 2: Controlled clinical trials of acupuncture for back pain

First author	Reference	Design	No.
Edelist	*Can Anaesth Soc J* 1976; 23: 303-306	RCT patient-and evaluator-blind	30
Yue	*Acupuncture Electrother Res* 1978;3:323-324	RCT evaluator-blind 3 parallel arms	23
Lopacz	*Neurol Neurochir Pol* 1979;13:405-409	RCT non-blind 2 parallel arms	34
Coan	Am J Chin Med 1980; 8:181-189	RCT non-blind 2 parallel arms	48
Gunn	Spine 1980; 5:279-291	RCT non-blind 2 parallel arms	46
Gallacchi	Schweiz med Wschr 1981; 111:1360-1366	RCT non-blind 8 parallel arms	~30
Duplan	Sem Hop Paris 1983;59: 3109-3114	RCT patient-and evaluator-blind 2 parallel arms	30
Macdonald	Ann R Coll Surg Engl 1983; 65:44-46	RCT patient – and evaluator-blind 2 parallel arms	16
Mendelson	Am J Med 1983;74:49-55	RCT patient – and evaluator-blind crossover	77
Lehmann	Pain 1986; 26:277-290	RCT non-blind 3 parallel arms	53
Garvey	Spine 1989; 14:962-964	RCT patient-and evaluator-blind 4 parallel arms	63
Thomas	Acta Anaesthesiol Scand 1994;38:63-69	RCT non-blind, voluntary crossover, with untreated controls	40

Acup = acupuncture; EA = electroacupuncture; NS = not significant; VAS = visual analogue scale.

Interventions	Endpoint	Main result
Formula EA vs sham acup	Evaluator's rating of improvement	No intergroup differences
Formula acup.vs sham acup vs physiotherapy	Pain, range of movement	Acup was superior to physiotherapy but not to sham
Formula acup + NaCl injection vs sham electrical stimulation	Global assessment by physician	Acup superior to controls (NS)
Individualised traditional acup. vs waiting-list controls	Pain score	Pain reduction: Acup 51%, controls 2%
Needling at muscle motor point (mean 7.9) + standard physiotherapy vs physiotherapy alone	Pain and work status	Needling superior to controls (P<0.01)
Formula acup vs 2 forms of sham acup vs 5 forms of laser acup	VAS for pain	All groups improved, no intergroup differences
Formula acup vs sham acup	Pain VAS on standing 10 minutes, and on resting	Acup superior to sham for severe pain
Superficial needling (±EA) vs sham TENS	VAS for pain, etc	Pain reduction greater after needling (P<0.01)
Formula acup vs lidocaine injections	VAS for pain	No significant difference between groups
Individualised EA vs TENS vs sham TENS; + education and exercise programme	VAS for pain and disability + physician's assessment	EA superior to TENS (NS); no difference between TENS and sham TENS
Trigger point needling vs vapocoolant spray + acupressure vs lidocaine injection vs lidocaine + steroid injection	Evaluator's rating of improvement	Needling and acupressure yielded the best results (NS)
Flexible formula acup vs low frequency EA vs high frequency LA by patient choice (average 6.8) vs waiting –list controls	Activity related to pain, mobility, verbal descriptors of pain, patient's assessment of condition	After 6 weeks all EA groups superior to untreated controls (P<0.05); after 6 months this was only the case for low frequency EA

Source: Ernst E (1999). Clinical effectiveness of acupuncture: an overview of systematic reviews. In E Ernst & A White (eds.) Acupuncture: a scientific appraisal. Oxford: Butterworth-Heinemann
Reprinted by permission of Butterworth-Heinemann

Table 3: Controlled trials of acupuncture for neck pain

First Author	Reference	Design	No.
Gallacchi	Schweiz Med Wschr 1981; 111(37): 1360-1366	RCT parallel groups	45
Coan	Am J Chin Med 1982; 9: 326-332	RCT parallel groups	30
Junnila	Am J Acupunct 1982; 10: 259-262	RCT parallel groups	44
Loy	Med J Aust 1983; 2: 32-34	RCT parallel groups	60
Petrie	Clin Exp Rheumatol 1983; 1: 333-335	RCT parallel groups	13
Emery	Br J Rheumatol 1986; 25: 132-133	RCT crossover	20
Kreczi	Acupunct Electrother Res 1986; 11: 207-216	RCT crossover (short term)	42
Petrie	Br J Rheumatol 1986; 25: 271-275	RCT parallel groups	25
Ceccherelli	Clin J Pain 1989; 5: 301-304	RCT parallel groups	27
Lundeberg	Pain Clinic 1991; 4: 155-161	RCT parallel groups (short-term)	58
Thomas	Am J Chin Med 1991; 19: 95-100	RCT crossover (short-term)	176
Kisiel	Sjukgymnasten 1996; 12: S24-S31	RCT parallel groups	19
David	Unpublished	RCT parallel groups	70
Irnich	Unpublished	RCT crossover	68

Acup = acupuncture; EA = electroacupuncture; OA = osteoarthritis; ROM = range of movement; stats = statistics; VAS = visual analogue scale.

Interventions (session)	Endpoint	Main result
Formula acup	Pain (VAS)	a) acup = sham
A) sham acup	No follow-up	b) acup = non-point
B) non-point needling		
Classical individual acup waiting list	Pain (hour/day)	Acup significant > nil
	Follow-up 3 months	
Formula acup	Pain (VAS)	
Sham: pricked with fingernail	Follow-up 1 month	Acup significant > sham
Points from list physiotherapy	ROM, pain relief percent	Acup 87% relief physiotherapy
(short-wave, traction)	Follow-up 6 weeks	54% relief no stats
Formula acup, sham TENS	Pain relief scale	Acup significant > sham TENS
	No follow up	
Formula + EA	Pain (VAS)	Acup = sham
sham: needle-prick only	No follow up	
Laser acup	Pain (VAS)	Laser significant > mock
Sham laser	Follow-up 24 hours	Laser up to 6 hours
		Laser = mock laser at 24 hours
Formula acup	Pain (VAS)	Acup = sham
Sham TENS	Follow-up 1 week	
Laser to tender + acup points	Pain (McGill)	Laser significant > placebo
sham laser	Follow-up 3 months	
A) formula, manual acup	Pain (VAS)	Acup = sham = EA 2Hz = EA
B) EA 2Hz	Follow-up 140 mins	80 Hz
C) EA 80 Hz		
D) superficial needling		
Formula acup	Sensory & affective	a) acup = superficial acup
A) superficial acup	pain (VAS)	b) acup = diazepam
B) diazepam	Follow-up 2 hours	c) acup sig > placebo diazepam
C) placebo diazepam		
Flexible formula acup, physiotherapy	Pain (VAS)	Acup = physiotherapy
	Follow-up 6 months	
Formula + tender points physiotherapy	Pain (VAS)	Acup = physiotherapy
	Follow-up 6 months	
Local and distant points from list	ROM, pain	
A) dry needling		a) acup slightly > dry needling
B) sham laser		b) acup significant > sham laser

Source: Ernst E (1999). Clinical effectiveness of acupuncture: an overview of systematic reviews. In E Ernst & A White (eds.) Acupuncture: a scientific appraisal. Oxford: Butterworth-Heinemann
Reprinted by permission of Butterworth-Heinemann

Table 4: Controlled trials of acupuncture for osteoarthritis

First author	Reference	Design	No.
Gaw	N Engl J Med 1975; 293: 375-378	RCT double-blind, sham-controlled	40 patients/ various sites
Coan	Am J Chin Med 1982; 9: 326-332	RCT	30 patients/ cervical
Junnila	Am J Acupunct 1982; 10: 341-347	Crossover trial, non-random, not blinded	32 patients/ large joints
Loy	Med J Aust 1983; 2: 32-34	Controlled clinical trial	60 patients cervical
Petrie	Clin Exp Rheumatol 1983; 1: 333-335	RCT	13 patients cervical
Petrie	Br J Rheumatol, 1986; 25: 271-275	RCT single-blind	25 patients cervical
Ammer	Wien Med Wochenschr 1988; 22: 566-569	Controlled clinical trial	14 patients/ knee
Petrou	Scand J Acupunct 1988; 3: 112-115	RCT, sham-controlled	31 patients/ knee
Dickens	Compl Med Res 1989; 3: 5-8	RCT single-blind	12 patients/ trapezio-metacarpal joint
Thomas	Am J Chin Med 1991; 14: 95-100	Randomised crossover trial	44 patients/ cervical
Christensen	Acta Anaesthesiol Scand 1992; 36: 519-525	RCT, single-blind	29 patients/ knee(s)
Takeda	Arthritis Care Res 1994; 7: 118-122	RCT, double-blind, sham-controlled	40 patients/ knee(s)
Fink	Forsch Kompl Med 1996: (abstract)	RCT, single-blind, sham-controlled	67 patients/ hip

RCT = randomised controlled trial; ROM = range of motion; TENS = transcutaneous nerve stimulation; VAS = visual analogue scale.

Source: Ernst E (1999). Clinical effectiveness of acupuncture: an overview of systematic reviews. In E Ernst & A White (eds.) Acupuncture: a scientific appraisal. Oxford: Butterworth-Heinemann
Reprinted by permission of Butterworth-Heinemann

Interventions	Endpoint	Main result
Formula acup vs acup at placebo points, once/week	Tenderness, subjective report	Both groups improved, no intergroup differences
Electroacup and moxibustion to traditional points (2-3/week for 12 weeks) vs no treatment controls	Pain	Acup group 40% pain reduction, controls 2% pain increase
Formula acup, individualised frequency of treatment vs piroxicam (20 mg/day), for 4 months	Pain by VAS	At end of treatment period significantly less pain in acup group. 2 months later effect sustained
Formula electroacup vs physiotherapy for 4 weeks	Subjective improvement and ROM	Acup group showed numerically better results
Formula acup vs sham TENS, twice weekly for 4 weeks	Pain	Significantly greater pain relief in acup group
Formula acup vs TENS for 4 weeks	Pain, function, analgesics use	At end of treatment period and at 1 month follow-up no intergroup differences
Formula acup vs physiotherapy for 4 weeks	Pain and other symptoms	Some improvement in both groups but significantly more with physiotherapy
Formula vs sham acup 3 times/week for 3 weeks	Pain by VAS	Significantly more improvement in real compared to sham acup
Formula acup vs sham TENS 3 times/week for 2 weeks	Pain	Acup was numerically superior
Formula vs sham acup, each session = 40 min, no. of sessions not mentioned	Pain by VAS	Both groups improved; no intergroup differences
Formula acup 2 times/week for 3 weeks vs no treatment group	Analgesic use, pain function (ROM)	All variable were significantly more improved in acup group
Formula vs sham acup 3 times/week for 3 weeks	2 validated pain rating scales, pain threshold at knee	Both groups improved, no intergroup differences
Formula vs sham acup	Pain by VAS, ROM	Both groups improved, no intergroup differences

Table 5: Systematic reviews of acupuncture for various indications

Authors	Indication	Studies included	Results
Vickers, 1996	Nausea and vomiting (all causes)	33 CCTs, 1932 subjects	27/29 positive; 4 negative when treatment given under anaesthetic
Murphy, 1998	Nausea of pregnancy	7 RCTs, 686 subjects	May afford relief, but possibly non-specific effect
Lee & Done, 1999	Post-operative nausea and vomiting	19 RCTs, 1679 subjects	Positive for early post-operative nausea and vomiting
Melchart et al., 1999	Recurrent headache	22 RCTs, 1042 subjects	Positive for migraine: inconclusive (positive trend) for tension headache
Ernst & White, 1999	Temporomandibular joint dysfunction	6 reports, 3 RCTs, 205 subjects	All positive but none controlled for placebo effect
Berman et al., 1999	Fibromyalgia	3 CCTs, 149 subjects. 4 cohort studies	Limited data suggest a positive effect
Park et al., 2000	Tinnitus	6 RCTs, 185 subjects	Acupuncture not demonstrated to be effective
Lautenschlaeger, 1997	Rheumatoid arthritis, spondylarthropathy, lupus etc.	17 studies of any design	Acupuncture cannot be recommended for these conditions
Linde et al., 2000	Asthma	7 RCTs, 174 subjects	Not possible to make any recommendations

Table 6: Controlled clinical trials of acupuncture for smoking cessation

First author	Reference	Design[1]	No.
Clavel	Rev Epidém Santé Publ 1992;40: 187-190	Sham-controlled, single-blind RCT 4 parallel groups	996
Gilbey	Am J Acupunct 1977; 5:239-247	Sham-controlled, single-blind RCT	92
Gillams	Practitioner 1984;228: 341-344	Sham –controlled, single-blind RCT 3 parallel groups	81
Lacroix	Ann Méd Interne 1977: 128:405-408	Sham controlled, single-blind RCT	117
Lagrue	Nouv Presse Méd 1977;9:966	Sham-controlled, single-blind RCT	154
Lamontagne	Can Med Assoc J 1980;5:787-790	Sham-controlled, single-blind RCT 3 parallel groups	75
Martin	N Z Med J 1981;93: 421-423	Sham-controlled, single-blind RCT 4 parallel groups	260
Parker	AM J Acupunct 1977; 5:363:366	Sham-controlled, single-blind RCT	41
Steiner	AM J Chin Med 1982; 10:107-121	Sham-controlled, single-blind RCT	22
Vandevenne	Sem Hôp Paris 1985; 61:2155-2160	Sham-controlled, single-blind RCT	200

[1] Two parallel groups unless stated otherwise
EA = electroacupuncture

Table 7: Controlled clinical trials of acupuncture for stroke

First author	Reference	Design	No.
Zou	Chin J Mod Dev Trad Med 1990; 10: 195-202	RCT, open	63 patients with cerebral infarction
Hu	Neuroepidemiology 1993; 12: 106-113	RCT, open	30 acute stroke patients
Johansson	Neurology 1993; 43: 2189-2192	RCT, open	78 subacute stroke patients
Li	Chen Tzu Yen Chiu Acu Res 1994; 19: 4-7	RCT, open	108 patients with stoke
Liang	J Trad Chin Med 1994; 14: 110-114	Controlled trial, open	101 patients with stroke
Sallström	Tidskrift Den Norske Laegefor 1995; 115: 2884-2887	RCT, open	45 subacute stroke patients

RCT = randomised controlled trial.
[1] Experimental groups received regular acupuncture in addition.

Interventions	Endpoint	Main result
A) Facial points B) Sham points both with nicotine or placebo gum	Cessation at 13 months	No significant difference between groups
A) Auricular points B) Sham points	Cessation at 3 months	No significant difference between groups
A) Auricular points B) Sham points C) Behaviour therapy	Cessation at 6 months	No significant difference between groups
A) Facial points B) Sham points	Cessation at 2 weeks	Acup significantly more effective than sham (P< 0.01)
A) Facial points B) Sham points	Cessation at 1 week	No significant difference between groups
A) Auricular acup B) Body acup C) Waiting list control	Cessation at 6 months	No significant difference between groups
A) Auricular points B) as 1 + EA C) sham points D) as 3 + EA	Cessation at 6 months	No significant difference between groups
A) Auricular points B) as 1 +EA C) sham points D) as 3 + EA	Cessation at 6 weeks	No significant difference between groups
A) Body + Auricular points B) Sham points	Cessation at 4 weeks	No significant difference between groups
A) Body + facial points B) Sham points	Cessation at 12 months	No significant difference between groups

Source: Ernst E (1999). Clinical effectiveness of acupuncture: an overview of systematic reviews.
In E Ernst & A White (eds.) Acupuncture: a scientific appraisal. Oxford: Butterworth-Heinemann
Reprinted by permission of Butterworth-Heinemann

Interventions[1]	Endpoint	Main result
'Calan' (5mg) 4 tablets/day	Functional recovery	'the therapeutic effect in the acup group was better'
Standard medical and rehabilitative treatment	Barthel index	experimental group had significantly less deficit on days 28 and 90
Standard medical and rehabilitative treatments	Barthel index, activities of daily living	experimental group had significantly better outcome at 1 and 3 months. Also better quality of life.
Standard medical care	Functional recovery	experimental group fared significantly better than controls
Information incomplete	Functional recovery	'the therapeutic effects were encouraging'
Standard medical and rehabilitative treatments	Motor function, activities of daily living	experimental group had better outcome and quality of life after 6 weeks

Source: Ernst E (1999). Clinical effectiveness of acupuncture: an overview of systematic reviews. In E Ernst & A White (eds.) Acupuncture: a scientific appraisal. Oxford: Butterworth-Heinemann
Reprinted by permission of Butterworth-Heinemann

Table 8: Controlled trials of acupuncture for dental pain

First author	Reference	Design	No.
Bakke	Scand J Dent Res 1976; 84:404-408	CCT	33 volunteers
Brandwein	Am J Acup 1976; 4:370-375	CCT	184 patients
Chapman	Pain 1976; 2:265-283	RCT observer and patient-blind	60 healthy volunteers
Chapman	Pain 1976; 3:213-227	CCT	20 healthy volunteers
Sung	Anesth Analg 1977; 56:473-478	RCT patient-blind, observer-blind	40 male patients
Taub	J Am Dent Assoc 1977; 95: 555-561	RCT patient-blind	39 patients
Taub	Oral Surg Oral Med Oral Pathol 1979; 48: 205-210	RCT patient-blind, evaluator-blind	51 patients
Lapeer	J Can Dent Assoc 1987; 6:479-480	RCT	18 patients
Chapman	Pain 1982; 12:319	CCT crossover	40 healthy volunteers
Hansson	Oral Surg 1987; 64:285-286	RCT	21 patients
Kitade	Int J Acup Electrother Res 1990;15:121-135	RCT patient-blind	56 patients
Ekblom	Pain 1991; 44:241-247	RCT	110 patients
Simmons	Anesth Prog 1993; 40: 14-19	RCT double-blind, sham-controlled	40 volunteers
Lao	Acupunct Med 1994; 12: 13-17	RCT patient-blind	10 patients
Scarsella	Acupunct Med 1994; 12: 75-77	CCT	200 patients
Lao	Oral Surg Oral Med Oral Pathol Oral Radiol Endod 1995; 79: 423-428	RCT patient-blind	19 patients

CCT = controlled clinical trial; RCT = randomised clinical trial.

Interventions	Endpoint	Main result
A) without acup B) manual acup C) electroacup D) TENS	Pain threshold	Significant increase of threshold with electroacup
A) lidocaine B) needle acup (manual + electrical stimulation) C) lidocaine + acup	Pain during operation	In A, 70% felt no pain, in B 27% and in C 83% (no formal test statistics)
A) needle acup B) TENS at acup point C) sham needle acup D) no treatment	Pain after painful dental stimuli	A and B showed a small but significant analgesic response
A) 80 min electroacup at facial sites (2Hz) B) no analgesic treatment	Pain threshold	187% increase of pain threshold after acup
A) sham acup + oral placebo B) sham acup + 60 mg codeine C) acup at 2 Hoku points + oral placebo D) acup at 2 Hoku points + 60 mg codeine	Pain intensity during 3 hours postoperatively	Significantly (P<0.01) pain relief in C vs A and in D vs B
A) trad acup B) sham acup	Pain during operation (rated on 5-point scale by patient)	Numerically less pain in A (no formal test statistics)
Electroacup at Hoku points vs sham acup	Pain rated on a 5-point scale by patient and dentist	No intergroup differences. Success rate near 100% in both groups.
Electroacup vs conventional analgesics administered postoperatively	Pain intensity + analgesic use	No intergroup differences
A) control session B) acup session	Pain after painful dental stimuli	Decreased pain during the B sessions
Preop formula acup: A) = no stimulation B) = manual stimulation C) = electrical stimulation D) = electrical stimulation also during surgery	Intraoperative pain by VAS + use of conventional analgesia	No intergroup differences reported. Only two patients tolerated extraction without conventional analgesia (and both reported severe pain)
A) trad acup + oral placebo vs B) trad acup + D-phenyl-alanine (B) (slows degradation of enkephalins)	Pain during surgery rated by patient after tooth extraction on a 4-point scale	In group A there were good or excellent results in 42%, in group B 78%. No test statistics
A) preoperative acup B) postoperative acup C) no acup (all received local anaesthetics)	Pain during operation, pain after operation analgesics	In A and B more pain after operation than C. In A more pain during operation and more analgesics consumption than C
A) auricular electroacup + saline i.v. B) auricular electroacup + naloxone i.v. C) sham-auricular acup + saline i.v. D) sham auricular acup + naloxone i.v.	Pain threshold	18% increase of pain threshold with real acup, effect was partly blocked by naloxone
Acup immediately after surgery vs sham acup	Pain intensity and time until onset of pain	Acup was associated with 57% reduction of pain intensity. Time until onset of pain was 212 min in acup and 65 min in control group
A) electroacup at Hegu point B) site-specific points in addition	VAS for pain	In B significantly less post-operative pain than A
A) postoperative needle acup B) postoperative sham acup	Time until moderate pain, pain intensity	In A less pain and longer pain-free period

Source: Ernst E (1999). Clinical effectiveness of acupuncture: an overview of systematic reviews. In E Ernst & A White (eds.) Acupuncture: a scientific appraisal. Oxford: Butterworth-Heinemann Reprinted by permission of Butterworth-Heinemann

3

Safety: a review of adverse reactions to acupuncture

Introduction

It has been assumed in the past that acupuncture poses no risk, or very little risk, to the patient, and being a natural and holistic therapy is safer than conventional medicine and drug therapy (MacPherson, 1999). However, with its growth in popularity in Western society came the need for evidence of its safety, and with that came reports of adverse events from around the world (Rampes and James, 1995; Ernst and White, 1997, 1999; Peuker and Filler, 1997). A review by Rampes and James (1995), after a search of two databases (Medline and AMED), identified only 216 instances of serious complications worldwide over a 20-year period. The authors concluded that considering that 3% of the adult population of the UK were found to have consulted acupuncturists in 1984, that is, approximately 1.7 million people (Fulder, 1988), these figures are reassuring, particularly as the growth in the number of acupuncturists in the UK in the past two years has been substantial (see Appendix III). The complications generally fall into three main areas, physical injuries, infections and other adverse reactions.

Physical injuries

The most serious adverse effect that can be incurred during acupuncture is unilateral or bilateral pneumothorax. Insertion of needles into the thorax, particularly the intercostal spaces, paraspinal areas and supraclavicular regions can result in the puncture of the pleura and the lung parenchyma, and is potentially fatal. Several cases have been documented, for example, Rampes and James (1995) discovered 32 reported cases worldwide over a 27-year period, whilst Rampes and Peuker (1999) conclude that approximately 100 cases can be found in scientific publications worldwide. A Norwegian study (Norheim and Fønnebø, 1996) estimated that pneumothorax might be seen once every 120 years in a full time acupuncture practice.

Other documented physical injuries include cardiovascular traumas (Schiff, 1965; Nieda *et al.*, 1973; Cheng, 1991; Hasegawa *et al.*, 1991; Halvoren *et al.*, 1995; Kataoka, 1997), deep vein thrombosis and localised nerve damage (Bensoussan and Myers, 1996). Traumas to the spinal cord during needle insertion or due to migration of retained needles have also been reported, although the majority of these cases are a result of the Japanese practice of 'Okibari' involving permanent deep needle insertion. This technique is neither taught nor practised in the West, although its side effects are frequently cited in the literature, adding to the confusion surrounding the issue of the safety of acupuncture (MacPherson, 1999).

Many of the injuries can be avoided by ensuring acupuncturists are fully trained in anatomy and physiology, with particular emphasis on teaching the location and depth of the major organs. Even the most basic first aid course has such a component.

Infections

The invasive nature of acupuncture lends itself to the spread of infection when not practised safely or hygienically. Acupuncture has been implicated in the transmission of hepatitis, HIV and various bacterial infections including septicaemia (Pierik, 1982). The British

Blood Transfusion Service lists acupuncture as a condition necessitating temporary deferral for twelve months after the completion of the treatment if performed by someone other than a registered medical practitioner or health professional, or a member of the British Acupuncture Council (BAcC). (For further information telephone 0845 7711711). Members of BAcC can provide their patients, who wish to donate blood, with certificates confirming that the treatment was provided by an acupuncturist registered with the organisation.

Reports in the UK in the late 1970s of viral hepatitis infections from acupuncture needles (CDSC, 1977; Boxall, 1978) were influential in encouraging practitioners to use sterile disposable needles and the situation improved (Rampes and Peuker, 1999). However, there have since been further reports, with Rampes and James (1995) listing 126 reported cases of viral hepatitis, and Norheim's 1996 review revealing 100 cases of acupuncture-related hepatitis B and C reported between 1981 and 1994. All reports have in common the fact that sterilising procedures were inadequate.

There is no definitive evidence to support any concern that acupuncture needles can spread the HIV virus (Rampes and Peuker, 1999). However, there have been three cases of individuals acquiring HIV who reportedly had no other risk factors for the virus, other than attending an acupuncture clinic (Vittecoq *et al.*, 1989a, Castro *et al.*, 1988). However, due to lack of information in these cases it cannot be proven that acupuncture was the causal factor (Chamberland *et al.*, 1989; Vittecoq *et al.*, 1989b), and there could have been some other undisclosed risk factors, such as sexual practice (MacPherson and Gould, 1998).

The Department of Health has issued advice to practitioners of complementary and alternative medicine on the precautions to take to avoid the theoretical risk of transmission of variant Creutzfeldt-Jakob

Disease (vCJD) (DoH, April 2000). They state that although there is currently no evidence to link any cases of vCJD to date with any surgical procedures or with transmission by blood, the Department cannot rule out a possible risk and so considers it prudent to take precautions to avoid this theoretical transmission wherever possible. Practitioners of acupuncture are specifically told to have regard to this advice, and are advised to ensure that any needles or studs that puncture the skin are used only once, in line with the guidelines issued by WHO (1999).

Inadequate or improper sterilisation techniques are a serious risk factor and this is recognised by acupuncture professional bodies, and reflected in their codes of practice. Transmission of infections can be avoided if all practitioners use only pre-sterile disposable needles rather than reusable needles that require sterilisation. As Norheim's (1996) review found, all the cases of hepatitis transmission had in common inadequate sterilisation procedures, and most of the adverse events were due to "insufficient basic medical knowledge, low hygiene standards and inadequate acupuncture education".

Other adverse reactions

A range of other adverse events has been documented which are perhaps less serious than those documented here. These include bleeding on withdrawal of the needle (Chung, 1980), bruising at the site of insertion (Redfearne, 1991; Tuke, 1979), depression, insomnia, increased pain, burns from moxibustion (Bensoussan and Myers, 1996), and fainting (Chen *et al.*, 1990; Rajanna, 1983; Verma and Khamesra, 1989). Cases of skin reaction to metals have also been described (Castelain *et al.*, 1987; Fisher 1976; Tanii *et al.*, 1991) which can be avoided by using stainless steel needles without chrome and nickel.

One of the most frequently reported side effects is drowsiness, which may have implications for those who drive following treatment. One study (Brattberg, 1986) found that 56% of patients would have been at risk of an accident had they driven after treatment. The author speculated that this drowsiness might be the result of a fall in blood pressure or blood sugar, or the release of endogenous opiates, but that it would be impossible to predict who would experience it. Hence it was advised that, as with medication which might induce fatigue, patients should be warned against driving a car immediately after receiving acupuncture treatment. The study did not mention patients' concurrent medication however, and whether such medication may have contributed to or enhanced acupuncture drowsiness (Rampes, 1998). The Acupuncture Association of Chartered Physiotherapists advises their members in their Code of Ethics and Practice to recommend to their patients that they should not drive after treatment, until they recover from any drowsiness.

The risk of indirect adverse events such as mis-diagnosis or risk of omission has been discussed (Ernst, 1995) and needs to be addressed since it has implications for training, practice and health care delivery mechanisms. Since the extent of the problem is difficult to quantify due to its very nature, precautionary measures must be taken to reduce the risk. Practitioners should receive sufficient training to enable them to know the jurisdiction of their practice and its limitations. This is essential in order to prevent the application of inappropriate treatments (BMA, 1993). Acupuncturists should also encourage their patients to inform their GPs that they are receiving acupuncture treatment. Australia's National Health and Medical Research Council (1989) proposed that the undetected presence of a serious pathology by a practitioner of acupuncture is probably the most important of risks. Mills (1996) advocates the provision of a level of orthodox diagnostic training equivalent to that received by medical practitioners to counteract this possibility. A system of quantifying the risk is required in order to end the current state of speculation.

Practitioners should consider the potential for interactions between adverse reactions to acupuncture and adverse reactions to orthodox drugs being taken at the time of treatment. For example, acupuncturists should have some awareness of drugs that cause drowsiness, since overall drowsiness experienced by the patient after acupuncture treatment may be exacerbated. The importance of acupuncture practitioners finding out their patients' medical histories and general practitioners knowing about their patients' use of acupuncture is paramount to the avoidance of such situations.

Contraindications of acupuncture

Acupuncture is contraindicated in a number of situations which practitioners should be well aware of, and include: when patients are taking anticoagulant medication, when press needles (for auricular acupuncture) are used in patients with prosthetic or damaged heart valves, or when patients with pacemakers receive electroacupuncture. Electroacupuncture is also contraindicated if there is lack of skin sensation and in case of impaired circulation, severe arterial disease, undiagnosed fever, or severe skin lesions (WHO, 1999). The WHO (1999) advises that acupuncture is only used during pregnancy with great caution since the needling and manipulation of certain points may induce strong uterine contractions. The report advises "traditionally, acupuncture, and moxibustion are contraindicated for puncture points on the lower abdomen and lumbosacral region during the first trimester. After the third month, points on the upper abdomen and lumbosacral region, and points which cause strong sensations should be avoided, together with ear acupuncture points that may also induce labour". The Organization lists pregnancy as a condition that is contraindicated by electroacupuncture.

Rampes (1998) advises particular caution when acupuncture involves points on the thorax and immunosuppressed patients, and identified general precautions, which are always necessary:

• Remember orthodox diagnostic skills

• Use sterile disposable needles

• Use aseptic technique with press needles

• Lie the patient down during treatment

• Advise patient to avoid driving after treatment

• Count needles before and after treatment

• Observe patients for bleeding.

Difficulties with the evaluation of adverse reaction reports

The system of reporting adverse reactions to drugs and treatment in orthodox medicine is an area which attracts a great deal of debate in the medical world, with concerns about under-reporting (Pierfitte *et al.*, 1999) and problems with spontaneous reporting. Hence, it is hardly surprising that there are issues surrounding the reporting of adverse reactions in acupuncture. A major problem with the adverse reaction case studies which characterise this field of work is that often they do not contain sufficient information with which to critically appraise them (Ernst, 1995). Ernst suggested that future case studies should contain details of:

- Which acupuncture techniques were used

- Who gave it

- The timing of the adverse reaction

- Its reversibility

- Confounding factors.

White *et al.*, (1997) described different methods which could be used to assess the incidence of adverse reactions in complementary medicine, ie systematic literature reviews, surveys of patients and practitioners, case control studies, case registers, spontaneous reporting and observational studies. They concluded that spontaneous reporting is the most powerful method available, and is used widely in post-marketing surveillance of drugs. Systematic literature reviews, as cited in this chapter, are dependent on current databases for their literature. However, these may not be complete due to under-reporting of minor injuries by practitioners due to the frequency of their occurrence, or of more significant injuries due to GPs' lack of knowledge that their patient received acupuncture (Norheim and Fønnebø, 1996). They also cannot be used to accurately estimate incidence, since the number of treatments given per year is unknown. A survey, using members of the British Medical Acupuncture Society, of adverse events is currently underway using the spontaneous reporting technique at the Department of Complementary Medicine in Exeter.

Aside from academic work to assess the occurrence of adverse events, it is important to consider what individual practitioners can do. Mills (1996) suggests that awareness needs to be raised among CAM practitioners, and recommends that the research departments of the professional CAM organisations establish adverse effect reporting schemes. The first stage of this, he suggests, would be to familiarise the practising members with the process, perhaps using the organisations' annual conferences to introduce the measure and develop and pilot an appropriate report format. Rampes (1998), on the other hand, recommends the establishment of a national database for acupuncture adverse reactions similar to the British Committee of Safety of Medicines system of reporting of drug adverse reactions. This would collect and evaluate all reports of reactions to acupuncture, disseminate results to practitioners, and could be extended to cover other CAM therapies.

MacPherson and Gould (1998) recommended that the acupuncture profession undertake a UK-wide study to examine the key risks and their frequency of occurrence, which could demonstrate that the profession is concerned and responsible, as well as being useful in helping to promote good practice in the areas of risk. The British Acupuncture Council is currently funding such a survey through the collation of data from the effects of approximately 30,000 treatments. It is being conducted and co-ordinated by the Foundation for Traditional Chinese Medicine in York and aims to estimate the frequency and severity of adverse reactions, both minor, transient reactions and more serious, significant responses. It involves 1,850 members of BAcC monitoring their work with patients through May 2000. Their results should be directly comparable to those obtained in the Exeter survey mentioned previously.

Adverse reactions to acupuncture in perspective

The US National Institutes of Health (1997) stated that "one of the advantages of acupuncture is that the incidence of adverse effects is substantially lower than that of many drugs or other accepted procedures for the same conditions". The difficulty of estimating the incidence of these reactions has been discussed, but nonetheless some researchers have attempted the calculation. Norheim and Fønnebø (1996) estimated that for each year of full time acupuncture practice in Norway, 0.21 complications would arise (complications were classified as mechanical organ injuries, infections, and other adverse effects, not including point-bleeding or small haematomas). Bensoussan and Myers' Australian study (1996) estimated that the average number of adverse events per year of full time Traditional Chinese Medicine practice was one every eight months. Umlauf's (1988) study of acupuncture over a period of 10 years in a Czechoslovakian hospital evaluated 139,988 acupuncture treatments and found 8.9% (approximately 12,459 treatments) resulted in adverse events (faintness, fainting, haematoma, pneumothorax and retained needles). Considering that the Medicines Control Agency receives approximately 17,000-18,000 UK reports of suspected adverse reactions to all medicines each year, of which 55% are serious and 3% are fatal (Hansard, 2000), the incidence of adverse reactions to acupuncture appears relatively low.

4
Education and training

Introduction

There are a variety of ways in which acupuncture can be taught and practised. Broadly speaking, a practitioner of traditional acupuncture will make an individual diagnosis by interpreting the patient's symptoms and signs according to Chinese theory and assessment of yin-yang energy status, and will then apply needles to specific 'points' to rebalance energy, or 'Qi'. However, they may often also incorporate elements of orthodox medical diagnosis, which constitute the curriculum of many TCM acupuncture courses. Adjunctive therapies, including moxibustion (burning of herbs), massage, prescription for Chinese herbs, and advice on lifestyle and diet, are commonly also given. A practitioner of 'Western-style' acupuncture will take a conventional medical history and perform an examination. Acupuncture will be regarded as one of a number of therapeutic options and rather than moving the 'life force' or Qi, brief needling, (perhaps with fewer needles) is intended to stimulate nerve endings, and stimulate the release of endogenous opioids and other neurotransmitters. Within agreed parameters, a certain amount of diversity in acupuncture training establishments is healthy in catering for the individual needs of students and the different approaches and expertise among the teaching staff.

Principles of CAM education

The BMA (1993) suggested certain broad principles which could be applied – albeit at different levels for different therapies – to all training programmes for persons who intend to use CAM. As a primary step, it is essential that each therapy should establish a core curriculum, setting out the basic competencies required for the practise of that therapy by all practitioners, medical and non-medical alike. Courses should be of credible duration and type, to provide competent practitioners. Good practice would also suggest that a minimum, 'core' basic science/medical curriculum should be compulsory for all practices claiming to have a therapeutic influence. This foundation course might include some basic knowledge of pharmacology and an appreciation of the hazards in removing patients from prescribed medication, for instance, in interrupting a course of antibiotics. Most fundamentally, such a basic course would instil in all practitioners understanding of the ways in which apparently innocent symptoms – often the common ones – can often be indicative of serious disease. This element of core 'medical' knowledge is associated with the need for therapists to establish the limits of their competence, and to be aware of when it is necessary to actively encourage the involvement of the patient's doctor (Box 1).

Secondly, a regulatory body for a given therapy should assume responsibility for the clinical and professional accreditation of training establishments, by assessing compliance with established minimum standards in a particular therapy. The accreditation status could be renewable, probably every five years. Agreement on minimum requirements of training to ensure competence is needed for different levels of practitioners.

Teaching acupuncture

Techniques and philosophies in acupuncture have been evolving for over 3,000 years in a wide range of countries and these diverse traditions have been reflected in the training provided in national colleges. Many schools of Traditional Chinese Medicine in the West teach acupuncture based on the 'twelve pulses' and the 'law of five elements'. Some current Chinese teaching can be based on much simpler forms of TCM and in many instances just local acupuncture points are used to treat pain and no attempt is made to evaluate or treat the underlying imbalances of 'vital energy'. Western science seeks to explain the possible effects of acupuncture in terms of effects on humoral mediation via the circulation of neuro-transmitters and other hormones in the cerebrospinal fluid and blood stream (Hopwood, 1993), whilst also recognising the value of the 'holistic approach'.

Acupuncture treatment is now very popular in the USA and it is estimated that 9-12 million patients visit acupuncturists each year for treatments that involve up to 120 million needles (Lao, 1996). American doctors, osteopaths and chiropractors may use acupuncture without any or only limited extra training, according to individual State law. Other practitioners require specific training and for about the past 20 years State law has required acupuncturists to be licensed according to criteria developed by an Acupuncture Examining Committee and subsequently the National Commission for the Certification of Acupuncturists (NCCA). The examinations consisted of both written and practical tests.

At the present time, anyone within the UK can use the title 'acupuncturist' and, in common with many other CAM therapies, acupuncture is not regulated by statute and there are a number of different organisations, colleges and so forth offering training, education or registration in the subject.

Box 1: Competencies that acupuncturists and other CAM therapists should be able to demonstrate (BMA, 1993)

Competencies for CAM therapists

- A sound knowledge of anatomy, physiology, pathology, basic medical therapeutics, and the principles of their own therapeutic modality. The practitioner must also have acquired a sufficient depth of knowledge of the principles of medicine and the pathological process of disease, and be aware of the physiological basis for their treatment and modality.

- The ability to collect relevant information from the taking of an appropriate case history and an examination of the patient enabling the practitioner to formulate an appropriate diagnosis and effective treatment plan, as well as the likely prognosis and any suitable prophylaxis.

- An ability to conduct and interpret a relevant clinical examination and use currently accepted clinical testing procedures as well as an ability to interpret any ancillary tests.

- In reaching a diagnosis, a practitioner must be able to show that he or she has thought differentially using a rationale based upon current knowledge of anatomy, physiology, and pathology, demonstrating that he or she has considered not only the potential contra-indications of treatment but also has an awareness that symptoms manifested by the patient may be emanating from a site or cause distant from the presenting problem, and may be indicative of serious underlying disease.

- The practitioner should demonstrate an awareness of the relevance of a patient's personal life history, including psychological aspects, inherited predispositions, previous medical history, life-style factors, and social and occupational background. This is particularly important so that the patient's own expectations will be considered in formulating a treatment plan.

- Practitioners should show an awareness of limits of competence and the scope of their particular therapy, together with a knowledge of absolute and relative contra-indications to therapy. With this goes the ability to recognise conditions where a particular treatment is inappropriate, and also when a patient is suffering from a condition that requires immediate referral to the patient's GP.

- They should show an awareness of the need to plan a particular course of treatment and be able to anticipate its effectiveness with the patient concerned. A practitioner should be able to communicate his or her findings, diagnosis, prognosis and prophylaxis, where appropriate, not only to the patient's GP but also to the patient, in such a way that the patient's own expectations are taken into consideration.

- Practitioners should show an awareness of the need to evaluate and monitor the patient's progress in line with the proposed treatment plan and an awareness that, if anticipated outcomes are not met, consideration should be given to referral to the appropriate agency.

The major acupuncture bodies listed by the University of Exeter (Mills and Peacock, 1997; Mills and Budd, 2000) are:

- The British Acupuncture Council

- The British Medical Acupuncture Society

- British Academy of Western Acupuncture

- The Acupuncture Association of Chartered Physiotherapists

- The Fook Sang Acupuncture and Chinese Herbal Practitioners Association

- The European Federation of Modern Acupuncture

- The Modern Acupuncture Association.

(See Appendix II)

British Acupuncture Accreditation Board (BAAB)

As a result of a joint initiative of the Council for Complementary and Alternative Medicine and the Council for Acupuncture (CCAM/CFA) in the UK, a structure for accrediting independent schools and colleges of acupuncture was developed, and in November 1990 the British Acupuncture Accreditation Board (BAAB) was formally established. The Council for Acupuncture became the British Acupuncture Council (BAcC), in 1995.

Important questions to be addressed in acupuncture training include:

- what constitutes minimum professional standards for new practitioners?

- what constitutes an acceptable standard for on-going practice?

- when is 'full competence' achieved?

- what professional monitoring or 'training input' is required in post-registration years?

- what are key training issues related to safety, referral and management of patients?

The core syllabus now published by the UK BAAB and supported by the British Acupuncture Council includes topics such as history taking, basic theory, knowledge of acupuncture points, methods of diagnosis and treatment principles and techniques, including issues of safety and sterile procedures, anatomy, physiology, and research methods. The BAAB also puts great emphasis on professional competencies. The aim of training should also be to "encourage the development of a reflective, research-minded practitioner with qualities of integrity, humanity, caring, trust, responsibility, respect and confidentiality" (Shifrin, 1995).

Acupuncture courses

A BMA survey of CAM bodies (1993) reflected that there was a considerable range of standards, aspirations, and levels of training for practitioners of CAM therapies. At one end of the spectrum, the *discrete clinical disciplines* require levels of training commensurate with the responsibilities such therapists have to patients in their care, and courses for such disciplines are now likely to be degree equivalents. A BMA survey of UK higher education establishments in 1996 revealed that over 100 modules or complete courses in CAM subjects were being provided in universities, medical schools and faculties of nursing (Morgan *et al.*, 1998). Little information, however, was provided about specific research projects or research infrastructure, and none related directly to acupuncture.

The BMA 1993 report recognised that particular skills need to be acquired in order to achieve competence in different therapies, and highlighted the General Medical Council's statement that a question of serious professional misconduct may arise by "a doctor persisting in unsupervised practice of a branch of medicine without having the appropriate knowledge and skill or having acquired the experience which is necessary". Therefore, doctors (and nurses, physiotherapists and other healthcare professionals) may undertake specialised training to provide them with the necessary skills to understand and/or carry out acupuncture or other CAM therapies. One provider of CAM treatment specified that treatment is "complementary to conventional medicine and not alternative" and that all staff are members of the appropriate state registered health professions (RLHH, 1997). The BMA recommended in *Complementary Medicine: New Approaches to Good Practice* (BMA, 1993) that all medically qualified practitioners who wish to carry out acupuncture (and indeed any CAM therapy) should undertake recognised training in that field.

University teaching

Acupuncture is now established as a degree course at Bachelor level in at least two UK universities, run over three or five years, with a higher degree Masters course available for qualified physiotherapists. Graduates should have spent considerable time gaining clinical experience with patients, together with a sound knowledge of basic medical sciences, point selection and research methodology. Colleges and other institutions offering acupuncture education and training are able to apply to the BAAB for the institution and/or courses to be accredited. The rigorous accreditation process should ensure that only those organisations complying substantially with 17 essential requirements achieve recognised status (BAAB, 1998). The assessment programme should ensure that each training establishment is externally monitored against known assessment criteria. It should be expected that acupuncture students from any training background, as well as those practising the other '*discrete clinical disciplines*', should be able to demonstrate the levels of competence recommended by the BMA (1993) (Box 1).

Acupuncture organisations

Medically qualified individuals can undertake part-time training (for example, short courses of up to five days duration or during weekends) provided by the British Medical Acupuncture Society (BMAS). Qualifications are awarded at basic, intermediate and advanced level and BMAS accreditation requires 100 hours of learning and a presentation of 100 fully documented cases. Full training and clinical experience in acupuncture leads to the Diploma in Medical Acupuncture. BMAS promotional literature confirms that teaching on the basic course is based on scientific explanations for acupuncture as far as possible, but it also involves traditional Chinese concepts "at a simple level, when there is still no Western explanation for the effects in particular disease".

The Acupuncture Association of Chartered Physiotherapists (AACP) provides four categories of membership, according to the degree of training undertaken. An 'advanced member' will be a fully qualified state registered physiotherapist who will have undertaken at least 200 hours of training – the AACP confirms that individuals in this category are likely to be practising Traditional Chinese Acupuncture, but also to be involved in research.

The British Acupuncture Council has provided substantive guidelines for acupuncture education for institutions wishing to be accredited by BAcC. Such courses require study over 3,600 hours, with 200 hours personal management of patients through all aspects of their treatment. Courses will include biomedical sciences, anatomy and safe needling, diagnosis of serious underlying pathology, ethics and practice management.

The British Academy of Western Acupuncture (BAWA) is affiliated with BMAS, and was founded "in order to promote, enhance and unify the practice of acupuncture in the UK". It aims to ensure a high standard of practice within the NHS and private sectors. Membership is open to those with "suitable medical qualifications" including medical doctors, physiotherapists, and registered general nurses with a minimum of three years post-graduate experience. There are two grades of membership, granted to graduates of the BAWA Education Department's Licentiate Course.

The Fook Sang Association is an independent body offering specialist professional training in scientific and traditional methods of Chinese acupuncture and herbal medicine 'as taught in China'. The organisation offers flexible prescriptions in natural Chinese herbal medicine, including Chinese Folk Medicine using 'genuine Chinese diagnosis'.

The European Federation of Modern Acupuncture is 'an umbrella organisation enabling training establishments to enter into dialogue on matters of training standards'. Individual membership level is dependent on the degree of training undertaken at basic, intermediate and advanced level. Practitioners practise 'modern acupuncture' using a variety of means to measure the activity of acupuncture points/meridians, prior to treatment. Electronic, electrical and bioresonance devices are commonly used.

Members of the Modern Acupuncture Association undertake acupuncture training, clinical and tutorial studies, together with bioresonance or Voll systems, clinical kinesiology and auricular therapy. Practitioners vary widely in their approach, from needling to electroacupuncture, to changing the electro-potential of points by touch.

While differences in the training requirements of the various organisations do to some extent reflect the prior educational background of the students, there is a need for a consensus on the minimum standards of training required for all potential acupuncture practitioners. As discussed earlier, this should encompass basic knowledge of anatomy and physiology, awareness of limitations of competence, and so forth.

An updated edition of the University of Exeter survey of CAM bodies (Mills and Budd, 2000) provides an important overview of the current status of practitioners, differentiating between those who work as statutory health professionals (mainly doctors and physiotherapists) and those who work primarily as specialist acupuncturists. As well as different regulatory concerns, the report comments that the former "sometimes take the view that acupuncture is a technique to complement their conventional practice rather than an autonomous therapy (this is reflected in their educational requirements)". (See Appendices II and III for more information about these organisations).

National guidelines for acupuncture training

With the increasing use of acupuncture, the need for a common language to facilitate communication in teaching, research, clinical practice and exchange of information became essential. The World Health Organization (WHO) convened a scientific group which approved a standard international nomenclature and published *Guidelines on Basic Training and Safety in Acupuncture in 1999*, (WHO 1999). This document considers:

• the use of acupuncture in national health systems

• levels of training

- training programmes

- safety

- the importance of disinfection, equipment sterilisation, etc

The WHO recommendations for acupuncture training programmes cover personnel at various levels, including:

- acupuncture practitioners intending to work in national health services, who would have completed secondary schooling, university entrance or equivalent (and covered 'the basic sciences')

- full training/limited training for qualified physicians

- limited training for primary health care personnel.

National occupational standards in CAM

In the UK, an independent national training organisation, *Healthwork UK*, is assessing training needs for some professions within the health care sector. Its declared aim with regard to CAM is to assist practitioners in each area of CAM to work together to set high standards of practice, ensure quality education and training, and promote effective self-regulation. They recommend the establishment of a single lead body for each therapy that should represent at least 80% of the CAM practitioners currently practising a particular therapy. So far, national occupational standards have been published in aromatherapy, hypnotherapy, reflexology and homoeopathy (Healthwork UK, 1999, 2000). Healthwork UK has entered into discussions with the key UK acupuncture organisations about education and training standards.

Summary

With such a diversity of acupuncture organisations and qualifications, there is a need for the acceptance of a core curriculum for practitioners, including aspects of anatomy and physiology, research methodology, acupuncture techniques, fundamentals of orthodox diagnosis, and ethics. The courses should be of a credible duration and type to provide competent practitioners, with the ability to equip the students with the core competencies outlined in Box 1.

5

Acupuncture in primary care

Introduction

Previous studies undertaken in a number of countries have investigated the use of complementary medicine as a treatment option by general practitioners (GPs). Researchers have examined the demographic details of GPs to discover whether there are any noticeable characteristics that influence CAM use. Younger GPs have demonstrated a more positive attitude towards CAM, more use of CAM, and greater inclination to refer their patients to CAM practitioners than their older colleagues (Visser and Peters, 1990; Berman *et al.*, 1998). It has also been suggested that they have greater interest in receiving training in at least one CAM therapy (Franklin, 1992) and to refer to non-medically qualified practitioners (Wharton and Lewith, 1986). The type of general practice has also been found by some to relate to the practice of CAM; Verhoef and Sutherland (1995) found that those GPs working alone were more likely to refer to CAM therapists than those in a group practice, as did Anderson and Anderson (1987). Practitioners working alone may be more individualistic and more likely to try unorthodox treatment options, or they may be subject to less peer influence. Gender differences have been reported by some (Verhoef and Sutherland, 1995; White *et al.*, 1997), but not by others (Hadley, 1988), while referral has been reported to be more likely if the GP has personally used CAM (Reilly, 1983).

Provision of CAM by GPs

In England, a large postal survey found that 21.3% of GPs had referred patients for CAM in the preceeding week, and that 44.8% had endorsed or recommended CAM in the same period (Thomas *et al.*, 1995). The authors estimated that 39.5% of GP practices in England provide access to some form of CAM for their NHS patients. Acupuncture is one of the most popular therapies with reports citing from 19.8% (Anderson and Anderson, 1987) to 66% (Perkin *et al.*, 1994) of GPs sampled suggesting acupuncture treatment to their patients and arranging the treatment for them. One study in the south-west of England found 8% of GPs surveyed had arranged for their patients to visit an acupuncturist in one week alone, 4.3% had given acupuncture treatment themselves and 19.3% had endorsed acupuncture treatment (White *et al.*, 1997). Conditions for which GPs arrange acupuncture treatment include chronic pain, general pain, asthma, musculoskeletal indications, headaches, smoking, obesity, and tenosynovitis (Reilly, 1983; Knipschild *et al.*, 1990; Franklin, 1992; Verhoef and Sutherland, 1995).

Reasons given by GPs for arranging treatment by complementary therapists for their patients include doctors' confidence in the practitioner or the therapy itself, with some GPs believing that the treatment involves ideas and methods from which the orthodox practices might benefit. Half of GPs in one study cited lack of response to conventional treatment, 21% cited patient preference or request, and a further 21% believed in the effectiveness of CAM for certain disorders (Visser and Peters, 1990). Reasons given by doctors for non-referral include lack of available information, lack of belief in its efficacy, or that the treatment was not discussed (Franklin, 1992). Ernst and White (1999a), however, conclude that in surveys of doctors conducted since 1990, usually over one half of the respondents "have a positive attitude or believe that acupuncture works".

In terms of which healthcare practitioners GPs prefer to provide the treatment to their patients, preference seems to lie with other medical practitioners or physiotherapists (Hadley, 1988; Visser and Petas, 1990), although 87% of doctors in one study supported the right of "lay persons" to practise CAM (Franklin, 1992). Fairly high numbers of GPs have reported discussing CAM options with their patients (Anderson and Anderson, 1987; Visser and Peter, 1990), although few doctors in a study of 461 GPs in south-west England reported feeling confident enough to discuss acupuncture with their patients (White *et al.*, 1997). Perkin *et al.* (1994) reported 68% of GPs' patients had requested referral for acupuncture.

GPs' knowledge about acupuncture

Interestingly, despite the relatively high numbers of GPs arranging for their patients to visit acupuncturists, GPs tend to rate their knowledge about the therapy as relatively poor — for example, 78% of GPs in Avon, England rated their knowledge as poor or very poor (Wharton and Lewith, 1986). Perkin *et al.* (1994) found that although 95% of GPs knew the principles of acupuncture, only 24% knew the qualifications of the practitioners. As the authors point out, this is significant since doctors have an obligation to know the potential benefits and harm of making such referrals and fundamental to this is an awareness of what constitutes a properly trained practitioner. In addition to this, the NHS Confederation (1997) found that whilst patients do not necessarily see the NHS as their provider of CAM treatment, they do see NHS health professionals as an information source for CAM. With low levels of knowledge, GPs may be unable to fulfil this patient expectation.

The majority of the doctors still regarded acupuncture as a useful therapy despite their limited knowledge, and a small number had received some training in it. These numbers varied between studies, ranging from 3% in the UK (Wharton and Lewith, 1986), to 12% in New Zealand (Hadley, 1988), to 20% in Canada (Verhoef and Sutherland, 1995). Greater numbers expressed the desire to receive some form of training in acupuncture (ranging from 6% to 50%), or in another CAM therapy.

These studies are open to criticism since many have been based on small samples which may not be representative of the GP population as a whole. Those that were conducted outside the UK cannot necessarily be applied to the UK situation, and UK studies were generally not nationwide. They have tended to concentrate on complementary and alternative medicine as a whole and have not focused on any specific therapy. The BMA Board of Science and Education carried out a postal questionnaire survey of GPs to address the 1998 BMA ARM resolution, and to establish to what extent acupuncture is being used within primary care services in the UK at the present time.

BMA survey – The use of acupuncture in primary care services

A random sample of 650 UK general practitioners was selected from the BMA GP members' database of 27,922, representing 1.6% of the GP population overall and 2.3% of BMA GP members. The GPs were sent a four-page questionnaire containing 31 questions in June 1999, and an initial response rate of 43% (n = 280) was obtained, which increased to 56% (n = 365) after sending a reminder to non-responders. Some respondents did not answer all of the questions; the percentages reported here were calculated from the varying number of responses provided to each question, and these numbers are indicated. For main questions the number of 'no replies' is stated. The time-scale used was whether the GP had *ever* used CAM, in particular acupuncture, in their treatment options.

Major aims of the survey were:

1. To determine the extent to which acupuncture services are now being offered to patients via primary care services in the UK

2. To investigate GP opinions on who should provide acupuncture treatment

3. To investigate reasons why GPs may not arrange acupuncture treatment for their patients

4. To investigate levels of knowledge and training of acupuncture among GPs

5. To assess GP attitudes towards the provision of acupuncture in the NHS.

A summary of the main results can be seen in the discussion section, page 77.

1. Extent of acupuncture services being offered to patients via primary care services in the UK

A large proportion of the responding GPs (58%; n = 208/358) reported that they had arranged CAM for their patients, with the most popular therapies being acupuncture (47%; n = 169), followed by osteopathy (30%) and homoeopathy (25%) (Figure 1). As well as these main therapies, some GPs specified arranging healing, massage, reflexology, clinical ecology, Bach Flower remedies, Bowen technique, and hypnotherapy. No significant differences in referral were found between age groups or gender. A significant, but small, number of the GPs (11%; n = 41) employed a complementary therapist in their practice, whilst 41% (n = 150) provided the services of a physiotherapist.

Figure 1: Percentage of GPs arranging specific CAM therapies for their patients (n = 358, no replies = 7/365)

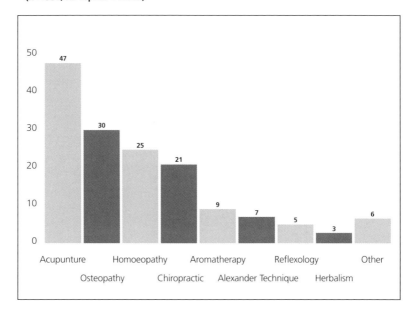

Location of acupuncture treatment provision

Of the 169 GPs arranging acupuncture treatment for their patients, 160 provided details of where it was administered. It was reported to be provided mainly within an orthodox healthcare setting such as the GPs' own surgeries (48%), in pain clinics (23%), physiotherapy departments (16%) and other NHS surgeries, clinics or non-homoeopathic hospitals (23%). Very few doctors arranged treatment at private homoeopathic clinics or hospitals (11%), NHS homoeopathic clinics or hospitals (4%), or in hospices (3%).

Conditions treated

Of the 169 GPs who reported arranging acupuncture treatment for their patients, 161 gave details of which medical conditions they did so for, shown in Figure 2. Pain relief and musculoskeletal disorders were the most frequently cited. Miscellaneous conditions which GPs treated using acupuncture included recurrent urinary infections, drug withdrawal, migraine, Bell's Palsy, hayfever and phantom limb syndrome, irritable bowel syndrome, anosmia (loss of sense of smell), and morning sickness.

Figure 2: Percentage of GPs arranging acupuncture treatment for different conditions (n = 161, no replies = 8/169)

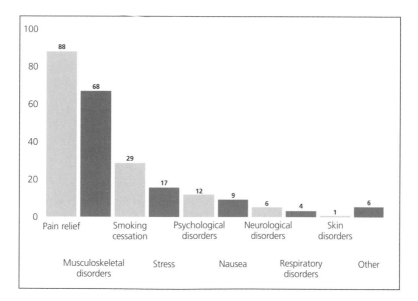

2. GPs' attitudes towards which healthcare professionals should provide acupuncture treatment

Attitudes towards which healthcare professionals should provide acupuncture treatment

The GPs who reported not having arranged treatment for their patients (n = 191) were asked which healthcare professionals they thought should provide the service. There was a significant bias in favour of registered medical practitioners, followed by physiotherapists and dentists. Less than half thought traditional Chinese Medical Practitioners should provide the service. The same question was asked of those GPs who had arranged acupuncture treatment, and they were found to have very similar attitudes. (Table 9). These attitudes and the actual referral practices as shown in Figure 3 differ markedly.

Which healthcare professionals actually provide the treatment

Of the 169 GPs who reported arranging acupuncture treatment for their patients, 162 gave details of which healthcare professionals provided the treatment. A number of GPs reported using more than one type of healthcare professional to provide acupuncture treatment for their patients, with the majority using the services of those already established in primary healthcare, another doctor (57%), a physiotherapist (24%), or themselves (15%). Although 19% stated that they arranged treatment by another complementary medicine practitioner, only 5% arranged treatment by a Traditional Chinese Medicine practitioner. A small number of doctors also reported referring to nurses, midwives, consultant anaesthetists, and healthcare workers in pain clinics, rheumatology clinics and drug clinics. (Figure 3).

Figure 3: Which healthcare professionals actually provide the acupuncture treatment?
(n = 162, no replies = 7/169)

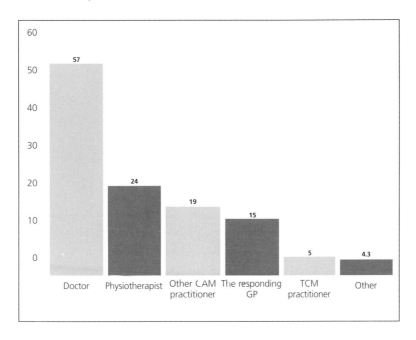

Many respondents commented on how they would choose an acupuncturist (n = 156, no replies = 13/169); a large number relied upon 'word of mouth' (48%). Only 2% consulted a professional acupuncture organisation, the same percentage chose through local advertising, while 23% said they assessed the qualifications or training of an individual themselves.

Table 9: GPs' views of which type of health professionals should provide acupuncture services

Type of health professional who should provide acupuncture treatment	% GPs not currently arranging acupuncture treatment n = 170, no replies = 21	% GPs arranging acupuncture treatment n = 153 no replies = 16
Doctors	79	85
Physiotherapists	71	75
Dentists	50	48
Nurses	47	52
Traditional Chinese Medicine practitioners	42	46
Midwives	39	47
Other complementary practitioners	38	46
Other	15	11

3. Reasons why GPs may not arrange acupuncture treatment for their patients

While acupuncture was reported to be the most widely used CAM treatment, just over half of the respondents had never used it in their treatment options (53%, n = 191/358). Three main reasons for this were cited by those who gave reasons (n = 188/191) (some GPs provided more than one reason):

• Lack of demand from the patients (63%)

• Lack of knowledge/information of services available (63%)

• Lack of guidelines to assess the competency of acupuncturists (45%) (See Figure 4 for further reasons).

Figure 4: GPs' reasons for not arranging acupuncture treatment for their patients (n = 188/191)

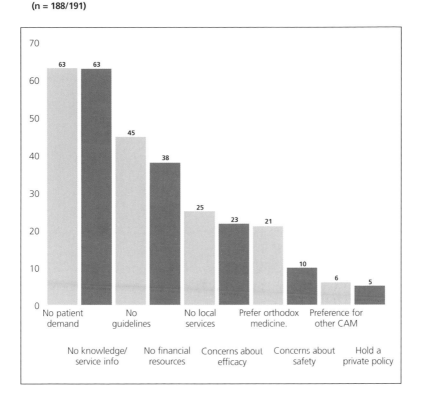

4. Levels of knowledge and training of acupuncture among GPs

The majority of GPs reported having either very little knowledge of complementary medicine (30%) or only knowing the basic details (52%). This was also true for their personal awareness of acupuncture (n = 364, no replies = 1/365), with 31% having very little knowledge, 53% knowing only the basic details, 6% knowing a considerable amount, and 10% felt they knew a lot about the subject. Most of the GPs who specified where they had received their knowledge and training about acupuncture (n = 63) reported that they had attended a course.

None reported receiving any acupuncture education at medical school. (Table 10).

Table 10: Source of GP knowledge about acupuncture (n = 63)

Where acupuncture training/knowledge was obtained	% of GPs	Number of GPs
Course	60	38
Seminar, lecture of informal conference	32	20
Informal advice from a colleague	27	17
Medical journals	21	13
Personal experience	19	12
Books	5	3
Tuition at medical school	0	0

The proportion of doctors who personally performed acupuncture for their patients (15%, n = 25/162) and those who considered themselves to have sufficient knowledge and training to perform it (12%, n = 41/354), closely corresponded.

Almost half of the GPs (46% n = 156/340) said they would like to receive some training in acupuncture in order to treat their patients in the future. This attitude was the same for those GPs who were already using acupuncture in their treatment options and those who were not, suggesting a large number of GPs are interested in the therapy regardless of whether they have made arrangements for their patients to receive it in the past.

Communication

Communication between patients and GPs appears mixed; in terms of patients initiating the discussion about acupuncture, the majority of GPs reported that their patients rarely (49%, n = 176/359) or only occasionally (37%, n = 134/359) do so. Only 6% of GPs said their patients frequently initiated the discussion, and 8% said patients had never raised the subject.

However, on uptake of the acupuncture treatment, communication between GP and patient is high, with only 3% (n = 5/160) of GPs stating that they never receive feedback from the patient on the efficacy of the treatment, and most (49%, n = 78/160) stating that they 'usually' receive feedback. In terms of communication between the GPs and the acupuncturists (n = 158, no replies = 11/169), the majority of GPs 'sometimes' liaise directly with the acupuncturist about the patient's treatment (36%) or 'usually' do (27%). Only 18% 'always' liaise with the acupuncturist and a similar number (19%) never do.

5. GPs' attitudes to the provision of acupuncture in the NHS

Overall, 79% (n = 265/336) of the GPs agreed that they would like to see acupuncture available on the NHS. Similar reasons for this belief were given by GPs who had not referred patients to an acupuncturist, as were given by those who had (Figure 5).

Figure 5: GPs' reasons for wanting acupuncture available on the NHS (n = 265 no replies = 29/365)

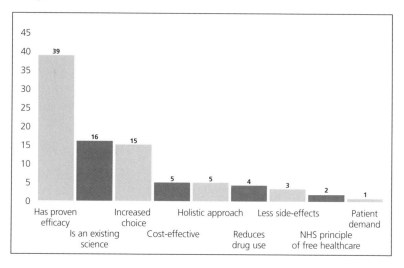

Of the 21% (n = 71/336) of doctors who felt that it would be inappropriate to make acupuncture available on the NHS, the principal reasons given were:

- lack of evidence (34%)

- lack of time and financial resources (54%)

- belief that it is a non-essential service (5%).

Discussion

The main findings are as follows:

- The results are based on the responses of 365 GPs (56% response rate)

- 58% of responders had arranged CAM for their patients

- 47% (n = 169) of responders had arranged acupuncture for their patients

- Almost half the acupuncture arranged was provided in the GP surgery

- 15% of GPs who had arranged acupuncture, provided it themselves. 57% used another doctor. 24% had used a physiotherapist and only 5% had used a TCM practitioner

- Acupuncture was most commonly arranged for pain relief and musculoskeletal disorders

- 97% of GPs who arranged acupuncture said they received feedback from their patients. Only 18% said that they always liaised with the acupuncturist following a referral

- Whether they had used acupuncture or not, responding GPs believed that doctors and physiotherapists were the most appropriate providers of acupuncture in primary care. However, almost half of all responding GPs believed that TCM acupuncturists were suitable providers

- GPs not using acupuncture cited lack of patient demand, lack of knowledge or information about services available, lack of guidelines to assess competency of acupuncturists, and lack of financial resources as the most common reasons for not doing so

- 16% of responding GPs said that they had "considerable knowledge" of acupuncture or "knew a lot about the subject"

- 46% of responding GPs said that they would like to receive further training in acupuncture in order to treat their own patients in the future

- 79% of responding GPs would like to see acupuncture provided in the NHS.

The survey has confirmed the findings of a previous study of general practitioners' use of CAM in England (Thomas *et al.*, 1995), indicating that a large proportion of general medical practitioners nationally are likely to be using CAM therapies in their treatment options, particularly acupuncture. The number of overall respondents is small, although compared to other studies that have investigated doctors' use of CAM, this number is relatively large. There is a possibility that there was response bias, since those GPs who use acupuncture in their treatment options may have perceived the subject as more salient than those GPs who did not, and hence had greater motivation to respond. This might, therefore, have influenced the findings for the GP group as a whole, although it is unlikely that it will have affected the results from the selective group of GPs arranging acupuncture.

As has been found previously, knowledge and training in CAM and acupuncture among the GP population was found to be low overall, while the desire for training for acupuncture was found to be generally high. This discrepancy needs to be addressed, perhaps through GP educational initiatives or continuing professional development, detailing conditions that can be treated with acupuncture, the evidence base of acupuncture, details of courses, qualifications, and so forth.

The NHS Confederation (1997) found that patients view NHS health professionals as an information source about CAM, although they did not view them as the providers of the treatment. However, only a small proportion of GPs in this study reported their patients initiating the discussion on acupuncture, and a large proportion of the GPs who gave reasons for not arranging acupuncture for their patients, stated there was no patient demand. With an estimated one in five people in the UK using some form of CAM (Ernst and White, 2000), their demand must be finding a different outlet. Those referrals and delegations documented here might very well be mainly professionally led rather than patient-led. It is possible that this situation has arisen because patients are concerned about their GPs' opinions of CAM and if this is found to be the case in any future research, ways to alleviate this concern should be sought. Mills and Budd (2000) speculate that if there was evidence that professionals from across the healthcare spectrum were engaging in "constructive debate about their relative roles", greater communication might be encouraged between patients and individual practitioners.

Communication between the GPs and their patients' acupuncturists was found to be mixed, with only a small proportion of GPs reporting that they always communicate with the acupuncturist. With no advice to guide GPs on choosing an acupuncturist and liasing with them, it is likely that this situation will remain the same. The opportunity to exchange details of their patients' medical histories, and hence inform each other in the event of an adverse event, may be missed.

The survey has revealed a discrepancy between the responding GPs' attitudes about which type of healthcare professional should in theory provide acupuncture treatment for their patients, and which type they recommend in practice. Almost half of those arranging acupuncture treatment felt Traditional Chinese Medicine practitioners should provide the treatment, but only 5% used such a practitioner in practice. A greater number of GPs were found to refer to medically qualified practitioners, rather than to other types of therapist, as has been found in previous studies. This could be due to the divide between Western and Traditional Chinese Medicine acupuncture itself. Most medically qualified acupuncturists practise Western acupuncture. The split between the Western approach to acupuncture and the traditional approach is one that tends to divide the medical profession and practitioners of acupuncture alike, and may prove difficult to resolve in a regulatory system. Future high quality research into both styles of practice may prove beneficial in this debate.

On the other hand, the discrepancy between the theory and practice of referral/delegation by the GPs could be due to the local level of service provision and the GPs' level of knowledge about it. One of the principal reasons GPs gave for not wishing to arrange acupuncture treatment for their patients was their lack of knowledge and information of services available. Considering that most GPs choose their acupuncturists by word of mouth, it perhaps isn't surprising that the vast majority arranged for treatment to be provided by their medical colleagues. Finally, one further consideration for this discrepancy is that when GPs refer to medically qualified acupuncturists, they are not required to assess their competence since their registration with the GMC is taken as evidence of that. However, in delegating to a non-medically qualified acupuncturist, the GP is responsible for assessing the training, qualifications and experience of that individual, a responsibility the GP might feel unable to fulfil adequately.

Regardless of whether they had ever arranged acupuncture treatment for their patients in the past, the majority of GPs believed that acupuncture should be available on the NHS. The principal reason given for this belief was that acupuncture has proven efficacy. However, as has been discussed in chapter two, so far evidence in favour of acupuncture has been found for only a small number of conditions. There is no strong evidence in favour of using acupuncture for smoking cessation, but a significant number of the GPs reported arranging acupuncture for their patients for this reason. There is therefore a need for dissemination of information to GPs. Other reasons given by the GPs for making acupuncture available on the NHS included increased choice for both patients and doctors, and a reduction in the use of prescription drugs. With such support for the move to make acupuncture available on the NHS, and such high numbers of GPs already using it in their treatment options, consideration should be given to ways of making it more easily accessible.

The 1986 BMA report *Alternative Therapy* commented, "Time, touch and compassion are all features of good medical practice. Alternative therapists do not have a unique claim on these aspects of healing, or a monopoly on their use". However, the pressures of a busy general practice may tend to limit the extent to which a medical practitioner can apply appropriate time-consuming skills, when on average only seven minutes of consultation time per doctor are available for each patient (Venning *et al.*, 2000). Further research into efficacy, safety and cost-effectiveness is crucial therefore, to the future development of CAM practice within primary care.

6

Future developments

Introduction

This report has confirmed that the provision of patient access to complementary medicine via primary care is widespread in the United Kingdom. Our survey reflects that over half of GPs nationally will consider arranging CAM treatment for their patients, and acupuncture is the most widely used therapy.

Efficacy, safety and training

Randomised controlled trials have demonstrated that acupuncture is more effective than sham acupuncture (or other experimental control interventions) for nausea and vomiting, back pain, dental pain and migraine. For other conditions, the evidence is uncertain. In terms of safety, few major adverse reactions to acupuncture treatment are reported in comparison to adverse reactions to orthodox interventions. For example, non-steroidal anti-inflammatory drugs (NSAIDs) prescribed for back pain and arthritis have been estimated to cause one death in every 1,200 patients who take them orally for at least 2 months. Extrapolated to an annual estimate, approximately 2,000 deaths occur in the UK which would not otherwise have taken place had the patients not taken the NSAIDs (Tramer *et al.*, 2000).

Opportunities for training in acupuncture, both for medically qualified and non-medically qualified individuals, have increased in recent years. The advent of validated degree courses and the emergence of CAM (elective) modules in the medical curriculum are evidence of greater acceptance, where previously attitudes may have been radically different. All acupuncture courses (eg undergraduate courses, weekend courses) should contain basic anatomy and physiology modules, with particular emphasis on the location and depth of major organs, and first aid skills.

Survey of GPs

Our snapshot survey of attitudes to CAM in general practice in the UK in 1999 has confirmed the findings of a previous study of general practitioners in England (Thomas *et al.*, 1995), indicating that large numbers of GPs are arranging CAM treatment for their patients. However, more GPs are now arranging acupuncture treatment (47% in 1999 versus 22% in 1995), with a preference for practitioners who are healthcare professionals, such as doctors or physiotherapists.

Overall levels of knowledge of acupuncture among GPs are low, although almost half of the BMA postal survey respondents indicated they would like to receive further training in the therapy in order to treat their patients in the future, regardless of whether they had ever arranged acupuncture treatment. Both these factors could be addressed by continuing professional development (CPD) opportunities. Those GPs who have not arranged acupuncture treatment for their patients cited reasons including lack of knowledge of local services, lack of guidelines and lack of patient demand.

The Medical Care Research Unit, in a major study of primary care CAM provision (Luff and Thomas, 1999), identified two key issues that underpin perceptions of the sustainability of complementary therapy services; credibility (cost-effectiveness and science base) and funding.

Funding

The provision of acupuncture treatment has flourished despite lack of widespread knowledge of its efficacy, lack of comprehensive guidelines for either GPs or patients, and without national regulatory and safety standards being in place for the practitioners themselves. One fundamental issue concerns funding, both for research and for service provision. In a primary care-led NHS, 86% of all health problems are managed entirely within primary care (DoH, 1999). The Government's current primary care research and development (R&D) strategy is summarised in *R&D in Primary Care National Working Group Report* (DoH, 1997), and was accompanied by a ministerial commitment to increase R&D spending on primary care research to £50 million by 2002-3. Figures show that only 0.08% of the NHS R&D funds were used in complementary medicine in 1996 (Ernst, 1996). Funding for service provision in the NHS based on evidence-based medicine depends on the availability of evidence of efficacy of the treatment. Large-scale trials are the best way to obtain this data, but are expensive to undertake. Research funds are urgently needed.

Sources of funding could include the NHS, Medical Research Council (MRC), via independent or joint initiatives, the Wellcome Trust, King's Fund, or perhaps The National Lottery. In fact, in February this year, the King's Fund awarded the Foundation for Integrated Medicine a substantial grant of £1 million to support their work on regulation. The European Commission's analysis of unconventional medicine (EC, 1998) recommended that those agencies, whether governmental or voluntary, who currently make funds available for research should be encouraged to allow for submissions from those working in unconventional medicine. Equally, CAM practitioners should ensure that their methodologies are in accordance with standards of good quality research. In the last five years the MRC has received six applications for grant support from researchers of CAM therapies, for relaxation techniques, herbal medicine, chiropractic, acupuncture, homoeopathy and hypnosis. All but one (a trial of chiropractic treatment for back pain in primary care) has failed to reach the competitive standard required for funding. Support is given to potential applicants in the form of advice on developing successful applications, which may include guidance from the Clinical Trials Manager on trial design, or in some cases, practical statistical help. The MRC have been involved in meetings with the Foundation for Integrated Medicine and also have a place on the Homoeopathic Trust Research Committee. The MRC and DoH have a joint initiative for research in primary care.

The NHS research and development budget for 2000-2001 will be over £448 million. There are no dedicated funds for research into CAM. Two grants have recently been awarded to researchers of acupuncture in the NHS Health Technology Assessment Programme (HTA). Both studies are pragmatic RCTs which also examine cost-effectiveness; one will evaluate the offer of acupuncture to patients with low back pain assessed as suitable for primary care management (mentioned in chapter 2), the other will evaluate acupuncture delivered by physiotherapists to patients with chronic migraine. The HTA programme aims to identify the most important gaps in the current knowledge that the NHS has about health technologies by soundings from key people and organisations, extracting research recommendations from high quality systematic reviews of research evidence, and using the Horizon Scanning Centre in the University of Birmingham. Criteria used in assessing research priorities include: what the benefits are from research in terms of reduced uncertainty, how long it might be before any benefits could be realised, and whether the assessment would be likely to offer value for money.

A separate NHS R&D programme, the Service Delivery and Organisation Programme, aims to "produce and promote the use of research evidence about how organisation and delivery of services can be improved to increase the quality of patient care, ensure better strategic outcomes and contribute to improved health" (DoH, May 2000). Such a programme could possibly provide funding for suitable research into the provision of acupuncture in primary care.

Further sources of funding for research include medical charities which spent 0.05% of their total research budget on CAM in 1999 (Ernst, 1999), and institutions which provide funding solely for CAM – the Blackie Foundation Trust, The Homoeopathic Trust, and the Foundation for Integrated Medicine. The 1993 BMA report suggested that many CAM therapists and organisations may not have the resources to develop adequate research infrastructure, and so funding from grant awarding medical research organisations appears essential to enable this development; as such funding has not been substantive in recent years the prospect of monies dedicated to encouraging and supporting high quality research should be considered. This would ensure funds are directed appropriately and would assist targeting and measurement of funding levels.

Cost-effectiveness

Cost-effectiveness will be an important issue for the potential future integration of acupuncture into the NHS. Very little is known about this issue (van Haselen, 1999), and there are few robust studies which have tackled it. Due to the lack of high technology in most CAM therapies, it is a common assumption that they will be less expensive than orthodox medicine. However, CAM consultations may take on average six times longer than GP consultations (Fulder and Munro, 1985). White *et al.* (1996) outlined four areas where cost savings might be made by using CAM: cost of drugs, visits to GP, secondary referrals and reducing adverse events of orthodox therapy. The analysis used to evaluate these savings can use the same factors that are used within orthodox medicine for economic evaluation; cost-comparison, cost-utility analysis, cost-effectiveness analysis, cost descriptions, and cost benefit analysis (White and Ernst, 2000). However, research conducted into the cost-effectiveness of CAM has tended not to follow such strong theoretical bases.

A systematic review of studies addressing the issue of economic analysis in CAM concluded that there is a lack of experimentally robust studies from which to draw conclusive evidence of differences between the costs and outcomes between complementary therapies and orthodox medicine (White and Ernst, 2000). The majority of studies which report evidence in favour of the CAM therapies, that is, evidence of reduced referral and treatment costs, are retrospective, while more rigorous and prospective studies suggest CAM is "an additional expense and does not substitute for orthodox care".

Economic analysis of acupuncture has suggested savings in reduced drug expenditure (Myers, 1991), reduced length of stay in hospital (Johansson, 1993) and reduced need for surgery for osteoarthritis of the knee (Christenssen *et al.*, 1992). Lindall (1999) concluded from a study of 65 patients suffering pain, that for selected patients, and when used by an appropriately qualified practitioner, acupuncture appeared to be a cost effective therapy for use in general practice, reducing the need for more expensive hospital referrals. An average minimum total saving for each patient was estimated at £232. However, due to methodological limitations the findings of these studies are not conclusive (White and Ernst, 2000). There is a need for high quality research into both the costs and benefits of acupuncture, particularly as primary care groups and trusts outline their health improvement plans in line with a remit to provide a cost-effective service.

Integration into the NHS

Over the last decade or so there have been major organisational and structural changes within primary care in the NHS. The late 1980s brought the introduction of fundholding (1989), and more recently primary care groups (PCGs) have been introduced in England (Local Health Groups in Wales, and Local Health Care Co-operatives in Scotland and Northern Ireland) (1999), which will eventually develop into primary care trusts (PCTs). One of the aims of fundholding was to give GPs greater awareness of, and responsibility for, their use of secondary care services, and the change was intended to lead to improved cost containment, cost-effectiveness, quality of care, patient choice and empowerment. There is consistent evidence that fundholding practices provided better access to secondary services, greater development of new practice-based services for patients, and reduced waiting lists (Samuel, 1992; Dowling, 1997). The provision of CAM was also facilitated by GP fundholding, since those fundholding practices were able to use the staff element of their budget to employ CAM practitioners. Non-fundholding GPs, on the other hand, were able to use their ancillary staff budget for this purpose, but at the expense of another member of staff. Local health commissions and authorities have sometimes used money for R&D or for waiting list initiatives to finance CAM provision (Zollman and Vickers, 1999).

With the NHS reforms in April 1999, uncertainty regarding the position of CAM in the NHS has emerged. PCGs are subcommittees of Health Authorities (HAs) and are dependent on them for some commissioning support. Their responsibilities include (NHSE 1998):

- to improve the health of, and address health inequalities in, their communities

- to develop primary care and community services (with an emphasis on reducing variability of services, developing clinical governance and increasing integration of primary and community care services)

- to advise on, or commission directly, a range of hospital services.

The introduction of the Health Improvement Programme (HImP) process will further assist PCGs and PCTs in strategic planning, taking account of locally determined needs, as well as national priorities. Concerns have been raised over whether CAM will be identified as a priority by significant numbers of GPs in individual PCGs; there is a risk that in the changeover from fundholding practices to PCGs, some established CAM services may be lost (Zollman and Vickers, 1999). With renewed emphasis on finance and efficiency, CAM therapies could be the first service to go.

Eventually PCGs will progress to Primary Care Trust status, which will be statutory bodies rather than subcommittees of Health Authorities. Being the sole commissioning bodies in the NHS, PCTs will be responsible for the commissioning of both primary and secondary care, and for the provision of primary care.

Models of provision of acupuncture in primary care

In order to facilitate the potential integration of acupuncture, and other CAM services, into the NHS, a greater understanding is required of possible models of provision. The Foundation for Integrated Medicine (1997), the Scottish Office Department of Health (1996) and the Medical Care Research Unit in Sheffield (Luff and Thomas, 1999) have examined methods used in general practice within England, Wales and Scotland. These include on-site provision by healthcare professionals, on-site provision by private practitioners, referral to NHS hospitals or complementary medicine referral centres, delegations to off-site private practitioners, and the use of networks of experienced medically qualified complementary practitioners (as has been established for homoeopathy at the Glasgow Homoeopathic Hospital). With the first Primary Care Trusts 'going live' this year, priority should be given to investigating nationally the optimum method of service provision.

Concerns have been raised about the limitations of CAM service provision on the NHS (Worth, 1995), and points have been highlighted which could possibly dilute the true potential of CAM when it is integrated. For example, Worth (1995) has warned that:

• The use of CAM therapies may be restricted to minor ailments or, at the other end of the scale, to chronic and incurable diseases where CAM is often viewed as the last resort

• CAM therapies sometimes may not show benefits as rapidly as conventional medicine, and doctors may resort too quickly to orthodox drugs if a condition does not improve within set time limits

• In addition, if CAM is subsumed within conventional medicine the opportunity to be "different" could be lost.

However, if the integration is accompanied by sufficient information and training opportunities for all involved, these risks may never materialise.

Guidance for Primary Care Groups and Trusts

GPs face potentially confusing guidance regarding their role in arranging for their patients to see CAM practitioners. Those GPs in our survey who did not believe it appropriate for acupuncture to be made available on the NHS (21%) cited reasons ranging from there being no proven efficacy and safety concerns, to there being no local services and a lack of information about acupuncture. The NHS Confederation report (1997) *Complementary Medicine in the NHS: managing the issues*, discovered four barriers to furthering complementary medicine usage which were consistently identified by healthcare purchasers, similar to the reasons GPs in our survey gave for not arranging acupuncture treatment for their patients. These were: lack of knowledge about therapists who should treat referred patients, lack of available funds, concern about the competence of practitioners, and lack of evidence. The doctors surveyed in the NHS Confederation report (1997) found an increase in the numbers of patients requesting information about CAM, although the patients did not necessarily view the NHS as their provider of CAM, but rather viewed the healthcare professionals as an information source. This patient perception adds to the importance of providing comprehensive information and guidance for general practitioners, particularly in light of our findings that 58% are arranging some form of CAM for their patients.

Guidelines for GPs should cover the following:

- Definition of acupuncture

- Where to find a local practitioner

- Details of what qualifications are expected of practitioners

- Details of GPs' medico-legal position

- Which conditions are likely to benefit from acupuncture

- Responsibilities in employing an acupuncturist – West Yorkshire Health Authority (1995) produced guidelines for GPs for the employment of complementary therapists in the NHS. Updated, nationally available guidance should now be drawn up

- Where to obtain further information, contacts, etc

- Codes of practice and ethics one should expect therapists to follow.

There is a need for greater consensus on the part of the Government, Department of Health, NHS Executive, the medical profession, and acupuncture organisations to provide guidelines and agree how acupuncture and other CAM services can be integrated into the UK healthcare system.

Recommendations

Integration of acupuncture into the NHS

1. Guidelines and recommendations on CAM use for GPs, practitioners, and patients are urgently needed, and the Department of Health should select key CAM therapies, including acupuncture, for appraisal by the National Institute for Clinical Excellence, for its third review programme in 2001-2002.

2. A general list of all acupuncturists, medically and non-medically qualified, should be produced and maintained by the NHS Executive, in order to facilitate the referral process for NHS doctors.

3. In light of the evidence supporting the use of acupuncture for back pain, dental pain, migraine, nausea and vomiting in appropriate patients, consideration should be given to the need for a policy, guidelines, and flexible mechanisms of making this treatment available to NHS patients. Health Authorities and Primary Care Groups/Trusts should give consideration to including acupuncture services in their Health Improvement Programmes.

Research and funding

4. Further research should be conducted into key issues including:

    - Investigating those other medical conditions that may be usefully treated by acupuncture, to ensure that patients who could gain the most benefit have access to acupuncture on the NHS

    - Investigating the cost-effectiveness of acupuncture treatment, with particular emphasis on the conditions that have so far been identified as possibly benefiting from the treatment (back pain, dental pain, migraine, nausea and vomiting).

5. Centrally provided research monies dedicated to CAM should be made available to grant-awarding medical research organisations. The establishment of groups who could help CAM researchers who do not have a research background should be encouraged. Established research groups should consider undertaking more collaborative work with CAM practitioners.

Regulation

6. The BMA commends the moves towards improving self-regulation made by the acupuncture organisations, and recommends that careful consideration should be given to the establishment of a single regulatory body, requiring the registration of all practitioners not currently subject to statutory regulation.

7. Acupuncture organisations should collaborate in creating a national surveillance system for the reporting of adverse events.

Communication

8. Strategies are needed to foster the relationship and communication between doctors, acupuncturists, and patients, such as:

    - An atmosphere of mutual respect between GPs and their patients regarding the use of acupuncture as a treatment option should be promoted to facilitate patients communicating the use of the therapy to their GPs

    - Doctors should ask about their patients' use of acupuncture and other CAM therapies whenever they obtain a medical history, and acupuncturists should recommend that their patients inform their GPs of their treatment

    - Acupuncturists should not alter the instructions or prescriptions given by a patient's medical practitioner without prior consultation or agreement with that doctor.

Training

9. Acupuncture should be included in any familiarisation course on CAM provided within the medical undergraduate curriculum.

10. Accredited postgraduate courses should be provided to inform GPs and other clinicians about acupuncture and the possible benefits for patients.

11. All acupuncture courses should have a core curriculum, with components including research methodology, information technology, statistics, fundamentals of orthodox medical diagnosis, ethics, and human anatomy and physiology, and should be subject

to external validation, with an examination board and external examiners.

12. All acupuncturists should be fully trained in infection control procedures, and immunisation against hepatitis B should be considered for the protection of themselves and their patients.

Appendix I

Glossary

Acupressure Similar to acupuncture, but instead of using needles, pressure is applied to the meridian points with fingers.

Acupuncture There are two main systems of acupuncture used – Western and Chinese acupuncture. The ancient Chinese system of medicine works on the theoretical belief that meridians, or energy channels, link inner organs and external points of the body. The acupuncturist applies fine steel needles at external points along these meridians (or sometimes burns tiny cones of herbal material over these points) to stimulate healing. In the Western system a non-traditional approach, based on modern concepts of neuroanatomy and physiology, is used.

Bach Flower Remedies Infusions made from extracts of flowers or wild plants diluted according to homoeopathic principles, which are taken internally to cure subtle emotional roots of disease.

Blinding The "blinding procedure" involves some of the people involved in a trial not knowing whether placebo or active treatment is being given – usually members of the study group. In a double-blind trial, both the patients and the researchers are 'blinded': In particular, the researchers do not know if they are giving an active treatment or a placebo. This is to avoid any subtle differences caused by their knowledge between the way they deal with patients in the active treatment group and the patients in the control group, and that could be detected by the recipients of the treatment. Blinding is removed only after the trial has run its course, and individual responses have been analysed.

Control A control group is used to establish whether or not a given intervention is the reason for an observed difference following treatment. This group is treated identically to the study group with the single exception that individuals do not receive the intervention.

Discrete clinical disciplines – homoeopathy, osteopathy, chiropractic, herbal medicine, acupuncture These are distinguished from other therapies by having more established foundations of training and have to differing degrees, established criteria of competence and professional standards and perhaps have the greatest potential for use in conjunction with orthodox structures of health care.

Ear acupuncture (Auricular therapy) Acupuncture solely applied to some of the many points in and around the ear, in order to affect other parts of the body.

Electroacupuncture A variation of acupuncture in which small electrical currents are applied to needles inserted into acupuncture points.

Endogenous An effect occurring without an obvious cause external to the body, and believed to originate from an internal cause.

The Five Elements This ascribes the qualities of Metal, Water, Wood, Fire and Earth to Qi in different processes of change associated with a particular season of the year. There are correspondences between one element and another, and energy flows between them in cycles. Each element represents a different human quality and different organs are associated with specific elements, as are senses and emotions.

Formula approach A standard formula is used to treat disorders based on a Western medical diagnosis. However, the points used are classical ones, and the formula may originally be derived from traditional Chinese ideas.

Healing May refer specifically to spiritual or psychic healing; spiritual healers lay their hands on the patient or may simply place their hands over the patient's body without touching it, in order to channel healing energies. Distance healing may be achieved through prayer or other kinds of thought processes and does not even require the presence of the recipient.

Hypnotherapy The therapeutic use of hypnotic suggestion, widely used to control or change undesirable behaviour patterns, and promote positive attitudes. Can also be used in the treatments of organic disorders and in pain relief.

Kinesiology A technique which studies the physics of body movement, in which muscular strength and balance at distant points of the body are used to determine the site and nature of a local impairment.

Laser acupuncture Low-level laser therapy is used to stimulate acupuncture points instead of needles. It is painless and therefore useful in children and those intolerant to needle insertion.

Massage Rubbing and kneading of areas of the body, normally using the hands.

Moxibustion A technique for applying heat by burning rolled cones of dried Artemisia (mugwort) over acupuncture points in order to affect the flow of energy (Qi) at those points, to prevent and treat diseases and disabilities.

Meridians In traditional Chinese medicine, these are considered to be invisible channels or pathways through the body along which energy (Qi) flows. There are said to be 14 main meridian channels that run to and from the hands and feet, and to the body and head, and along these the acupuncture points are found.

Neurotransmitters/neuromodulators Chemical messengers from nerve endings which mediate or modulate the transmission of impulses in the nervous system. These include noradrenaline, dopamine, serotonin, acetylcholine, GABA (gamma aminobutyric acid), NMDA (N-methyl-D-aspartate), endogenous opioids and many others.

Placebo Latin term meaning, 'I will please' - placebo is an inert substance or a non-effective treatment, but the person receiving it does not know this. For example, in drug trials all subjects receive a pill, but only in the study group does the pill contain the active substance. Placebo control is important in research, because when any form of therapy is offered, a large proportion of patients will report improvement based on the belief that the treatment will benefit them.

Qi Chinese term for the universal energy underlying the physical universe. The philosophy considers that bodies are made up of Qi, animated by it, needing a free flow of Qi for good health; acupuncture enhances the Qi of a meridian and restores and maintains health.

Randomisation All subjects in a trial should have an equal chance of being assigned to any groups that exist, and so must be allocated at random.

Reflexology Considers that different areas of the feet are held to correspond to other parts of the body through a system of internal connections. Massage of the appropriate area of the foot is believed to stimulate healing in the corresponding organ or part of the body.

Sham acupuncture Includes a range of control techniques such as needling at non-acupuncture points or inappropriate points, or in using non-invasive needling techniques.

TENS (transcutaneous electric nerve stimulation) Stimulation of body tissue with pulses of low-voltage electricity for pain relief.

Trigger points These tender points (or myofascial trigger points) are important in the causation of musculoskeletal pain.

Yin and Yang Negative and positive polarisations of life energy (Qi), considered by practitioners of Traditional Chinese Medicine to be contained within everything in varying proportions.

Appendix II

Acupuncture organisations

British Academy of Western Acupuncture
12 Poulton Green Close
Spital
Wirral CH63 9FS
Tel. 0151 608 0753 or 0151 343 9168

The British Acupuncture Council
63 Jeddo Road
London
W12 9HQ
Tel. 020 8735 0400

European Federation of Modern Acupuncture
59 Telford Crescent
Leigh
Lancs WN7 5LY
Tel. 01942 678 092

Fook Sang Acupuncture and Chinese Herbal Practitioners Association
590 Wokingham Road
Earley
Reading
Berks RG6 7HN
Tel. 0118 966 5454

The Modern Acupuncture Association
106 Higher Lane
Rainford
St Helens
Merseyside WAll 8AZ
Tel. 01744 883 737

Acupuncture Association of Chartered Physiotherapists
18 Woodlands Close
Dibden Purlieu
Southampton S045 4JG
Tel. 023 8084 5901

British Medical Acupuncture Society
Newton House
12 Marbury House
Whitley
Warrington
Cheshire WA4 4QW
Tel. 01925 730 727

Appendix III

The following report on the current position of acupuncture in the UK is reproduced with permission from *Professional Organisation of Complementary and Alternative Medicine in the United Kingdom 2000*, published by the Centre for Complementary Health Studies at the University of Exeter.

Further details of the Centre's work and copies of the report are available from:

Simon Mills, Director,
The Centre for Complementary Health Studies,
University of Exeter, Amory Building, Rennes Drive,
Exeter, EX4 4RJ
Tel: 01392 264 498

Acupuncture

There are two broad groups of practitioners of acupuncture in the UK, those who work as statutory health professionals and those who work primarily as specialist acupuncturists. The former include mainly doctors or physiotherapists: as well as different regulatory concerns they sometimes take the view that acupuncture is a technique to complement their conventional practice rather than an autonomous therapy (this is reflected in their educational requirements).

Of those whose members are primarily specialist acupuncturists, by far the largest group is the British Acupuncture Council (BAcC) which represents a unification of five professional groups established from the early 1960s. The BAcC has led the way among complementary professions in establishing verifiable standards of education for their profession. They are associated with the British Acupuncture Accreditation Board which, under an independent chair, works with the relevant training colleges to set and audit standards of education and training. The accreditation process is inclusive and other organisations may become involved in the future.

Of the other groups, calculations for the whole sector have had to leave out the position of the Fook Sang Association, which has a policy of not providing details about its membership. The EFMA has been established recently as an umbrella organisation with the Society of Electrotherapists and the Auricular Association of Great Britain as members; these practise modern techniques rather than traditional acupuncture.

In the case of the acupuncture professions, there is likely to be a relatively clear demarcation between the different professional groups. Overlap in membership is likely to be minimal.

Respondent Organisations were as follows:

	Year Established	Number of Practitioners
Organisations		
Complementary practitioners		
Modern Acupuncture Association (MAA)	1981	30
Fook Sang Acupuncture & Chinese Herbal		
Practitioners Association (FSACHPA)	1983	*not provided*
British Acupuncture Council (BAcC)	1995	2020
European Federation of		
Modern Acupuncture (EFMA)	1995	*not provided*
Subtotal		**2050**
Statutory health practitioners		
British Academy of		
Western Acupuncture (BAWA)	1976	250
British Medical Acupuncture Society (BMAS)	1980	1680
Acupuncture Assoc of		
Chartered Physiotherapists (AACP)	1984	1600
Subtotal		**3530**
TOTAL practising acupuncture		**5580**

Growth in previous two years

Complementary practitioners   36%   Statutory health practitioners   51%

Proportion of acupuncturists in organisations made up largely of *complementary practitioners* that:

- are registering bodies   the great majority
- obtain funding mainly through subscriptions   ALL
- have an elected council   ALL
- have paid administrative staff   the great majority
- use a formal accreditation process to screen membership   the great majority
- require members to graduate from a recognised college   ALL
- require continuing professional education   a small minority
- publish a professional register   ALL
- publish codes of ethics/practice   ALL
- publish formal complaints procedures freely available to the public   the great majority
- publish disciplinary codes and sanctions   the great majority
- require/provide professional indemnity and public liability insurance   ALL

Education requirements for membership   1200 hours (BAcC)

Update 1997-99

The BAcC has a new professional Chief Executive, a new core curriculum and is revising its codes of ethics and practice; it has set up a university-based Acupuncture Research Resource Centre to encourage undergraduate and postgraduate research.

Disciplinary sanctions 1997-99

There have been at least three practitioners struck off their register and more than ten warnings issued.

Summary responses from the organisations to other questions:

- **Willingness to increase disclosure of administrative affairs to the public**

  Great majority willing

- **Willingness to increase public representation on executive councils**

  Great majority willing

- **Likelihood of members proceeding in treatments without a doctor having seen the patient for those symptoms**

  Likely

- **Consider treatments combine well with conventional medical treatment**

  There were a range of opinions with a tendency to agreement

- **Views about regulation**

  The BAcC is due to have a referendum of its membership in May 2000; until it has that result, it will not formally take a position; the FSACHPA considers that a system of voluntary self-regulation would be preferable to a statutory route; MAA contains other practitioners among its membership and has no single position for acupuncture.

Proportion of acupuncturists in organisations with membership made up largely of *statutorily-registered practitioners* that:

- are registering bodies   ALL
- obtain funding mainly through subscriptions   ALL
- have an elected council   ALL
- have paid administrative staff   ALL
- use a formal accreditation process to screen membership   ALL
- require members to graduate from a recognised college   ALL
- require continuing professional education   ALL
- publish a professional register   ALL
- publish codes of ethics/practice   ALL
- publish formal complaints procedures freely available to the public   BMAS
- publish disciplinary codes and sanctions   NONE
- require/provide professional indemnity and public liability insurance   ALL

Education requirements for membership

Hours: 200(BAWA), 100(BMAS), 80(AACP)

Update 1997-99

The BMAS has a new Chief Executive Officer and a new accreditation procedure for entry into membership; the AACP has increased its entry requirement to 80 hours specialist acupuncture training and has developed an MSc degree programme.

Disciplinary sanctions 1997-99

There have been at least two struck off, one suspension and imposed conditions of practice; at least two letters of warning.

Summary responses from the organisations to other questions:

- **Willingness to increase disclosure of administrative affairs to the public**

  BMAS: "already full disclosure"; BAWA and AACP: willing

- **Willingness to increase public representation on executive councils**

  BMAS : conditionally willing; BAWA and AACP: willing

- **Likelihood of members proceeding in treatments without a doctor having seen the patient for those symptoms**

  Mostly unlikely

- **Consider treatments combine well with conventional medical treatment**

  In all cases

- **Views about regulation**

  Members already statutorily registered; however for the views of the BMAS, see below.

A common standard for acupuncture? Moves towards consensus

The formation of the BAcC continues to lead the agenda for complementary acupuncture practitioners. There have been occasional meetings between the BAcC and the BMAS and AACP. The MAA and FSACHPA remain separate. The BMAS sees a formal separation of "medical" and "traditional" acupuncturists and some distinction, therefore, in the regulatory development of the two streams; however, it has affiliated with the AACP and BAWA.

References

Anderson E and Anderson P. General practitioners and alternative medicine. *Journal of the Royal College of General Practitioners* 1987;37:52-5

Bensoussan A and Myers SP. *Towards a safer choice: the practice of traditional Chinese medicine in Australia*. Faculty of Health, University of Western Sydney: Macarthur, 1996

Berman BM, Singh BB, Hartnoll SM, Singh BK, and Reilly D. Primary care physicians and complementary-alternative medicine: training, attitudes and practice patterns. *Journal of American Board of Family Practitioners* 1998;11:272-81

Berman BM, Ezzo J, Hadhazy V and Swyers JP. Is acupuncture effective in the treatment of fibromyalgia? [Review] [25 refs]. *Journal of Family Practice* 1999;48:213-8

Black N, Boswell D, Gray A, Murphy S and Popay J. *Health and Disease: A Reader*. Milton Keynes: Oxford University Press, 1984

Black N. Why we need observational studies to evaluate the effectiveness of healthcare. *British Medical Journal* 1996;312:1215-8

Boxall EH. Acupuncture hepatitis in the West Midlands, 1977. *Journal of Medical Virology* 1978;2:377-9

Brattberg G. Acupuncture treatments: a traffic hazard? *American Journal of Acupuncture* 1986;14:265-7

British Acupuncture Accreditation Board. *Accreditation Handbook – Third Edition*. London: BAAB, 1998

British Medical Association. *Alternative Therapy*. London: BMA, 1986

British Medical Association. *Complementary Medicine: New approaches to Good Practice*. Oxford: Oxford University Press, 1993

Bruce DG, Golding JF, Hockenhull N and Pethybridge RJ. Acupressure and motion sickness. *Aviation, Space and Environmental Medicine* 1990;61:361-5

Castelain M, Castelain PY and Ricciardi R. Contact dermatitis to acupuncture needles. *Contact dermatitis* 1987;16:44

Castro KG, Lifson AR, White CR, Bush TJ, Chamberland ME, Lekatsas AM and Jaffe HW. Investigations of AIDS patients with no previously identified risk factors. *Journal of the American Medical Association* 1988;259:1339-42

Chamberland ME, Conley LJ and Buehler JW. Unusual modes of HIV transmission. *New England Journal of Medicine* 1989;321:1476

Chan K and Lee H. (eds) *The Way Forward for Chinese Medicine*. Reading: Harwood Academic Publishers, in press

Chen F, Hwang S, Lee H, Yang H and Chung C. Clinical study of syncope during acupuncture treatment. *Acupuncture Electrotherapy Research* 1990;15:107-19

Cheng TO. Pericardial effusion from self inserted needle in the heart. *European Heart Journal* 1991;12:958

Cheung L, Li P and Wong C. (eds) *Mechanisms of Acupuncture Therapy and Clinical Case Studies*. Reading: Harwood Academic Publishers, in press

Christenssen BV, Iuhl IU, Vilbek H, Bülow H-H, Dreijer NC and Rasmussen HF. Acupuncture treatment of severe osteoarthritis: A long-term study. *Acta anaesthesiologica Scandinavica* 1992;36:519-25

Chung C. Common errors and complications in acupuncture treatment. *Acupuncture Research Quarterly* 1980;4:51-8

Clinical Standards Advisory Group. *Services for patients with pain*. London: Department of Health,1999

Cochrane AL. Effectiveness and Efficiency. In: Black N, Boswell D, Gray A, Murphy S, Popay J (eds). *Health and disease – a reader*. Open University Press: Milton Keynes, 1984

Communicable Diseases Surveillance Centre of the PHLS. Acupuncture associated hepatitis in the West Midlands in 1977 [News] *British Medical Journal* 1977;2:1610

Department of Health. *NHS R&D Strategic Review Primary Care: Report of topic working group June 1999*. Summary on www.doh.gov.uk/research/report.htm

Department of Health. *Variant Creutzfeldt-Jakob Disease (vCJD): Advice to practitioners of complementary and alternative medicine,* April 2000 – at www.doh.gov.uk/pdfs/vcjdadvice.pdf

Department of Health. *NHS R&D – Organisation and Delivery,* May 2000 – at www.doh.gov.uk/research/rd3/nhsrandd/organisation.htm

Dowling B. Effect of fund holding on waiting times: database study. *British Medical Journal* 1997;315:290-2

Eisenberg DM, Kessler RC, Foster C, Norlock FE, Calkins DR and Delbanco TL. Unconventional medicine in the United States: prevalence, costs, and patterns of use. *New England Journal of Medicine* 1993;328:246-52

Eisenberg DM, Roger BD, Ettner SL, Appel S, Wilkey S, Van Rompay M and Kessler RC. Trends in alternative medicine use in the United States, 1990-1997. *JAMA* 1998;280:1569-75

Ernst E. The risks of acupuncture. *International Journal of Risk Safety Medicine* 1995;6:179-86

Ernst E. *Competence in complementary medicine.* Complementary Therapies in Medicine 1995;3:6-8

Ernst E. Regulating complementary medicine. Only 0.08% of funding for research in NHS goes to complementary medicine. *British Medical Journal* 1996;313:882

Ernst E. Acupuncture as a symptomatic treatment of osteoarthritis – a systematic review. *Scandinavian Journal of Rheumatology* 1997a;26:444-7

Ernst E. Acupuncture/acupressure for weight reduction? A systematic review. *Wiener Klinische Wochenschrift* 1997b;109:60-2

Ernst E. Funding research into complementary medicine: the situation in Britain. *Complementary Therapies in Medicine* 1999;7:250-3

Ernst E and Pittler MH. The effectiveness of acupuncture in treating acute dental pain: a systematic review. *British Dental Journal* 1998;184:443-7

Ernst E and White AR. Acupuncture as an adjuvant therapy in stroke rehabilitation? Wiener Medizinische Wochenschrift 1996;146:556-8

Ernst E and White A. Life-threatening adverse reactions of acupuncture? A systematic review. *Pain* 1997;71:123-6

Ernst E and White AR. Acupuncture for back pain: a meta-analysis of randomised controlled trials. *Archives of Internal Medicine* 1998;158:2235-41

Ernst E and White A. *Acupuncture: A scientific appraisal.* Oxford: Butterworth-Heinemann, 1999a

Ernst E and White AR. Acupuncture as a treatment for temporomandibular joint dysfunction: a systematic review of randomised trials. *Archives of Otolaryngology – Head & Neck Surgery* 1999b;125:269-72

Ernst E and White A. The BBC survey of complementary medicine use in the UK. *Complementary Therapies in Medicine* 2000;8:32-6

European Commission. *COST Action B4: Unconventional Medicine – Final report of the management committee 1993-98.* Luxembourg: Office for Official Publications of European Communities, 1998

European Committee for Homoeopathy. *A strategy for research in homeopathy: assessing the value of homeopathy for health care in Europe.* Rotterham: De Kruisff, 1997

Filshie J and White A. *Medical Acupuncture: a Western scientific approach.* Edinburgh: Churchill Livingstone, 1998

Fisher AA. Allergic dermatitis from acupuncture needles. *Cutis* 1976;38:226

Foundation for Integrated Medicine. *Integrated healthcare: a way forward for the next five years?* London: FIM, 1997

Franklin D. Medical practitioners' attitudes to complementary medicine. *Complementary Medical Research* 1992;6:69-71

Fulder S. *The Handbook of Complementary Medicine.* New York: Oxford University Press, 1988

Fulder S and Munro R. Complementary medicine in the United Kingdom: patients, practitioners, and consultations. *Lancet* 1985;2:542-5

Gahlinger PM. Motion Sickness: How to help your patients avoid travel travail. *Postgraduate Medicine* 1999;106:177-84

General Medical Services Committee. *Your choices for the future: results of the GMSC survey.* London: Electoral Reform Society, 1992

General Medical Council. *Tomorrow's Doctors: Recommendations on Undergraduate Medical Education.* London: GMC, 1993

General Medical Council. *Good Medical Practice.* London: GMC, 1998

Gosman-Hedstroem G, Claesson L, Klingenstierna U, Carlsson J, Olausson B, Frizell M *et al.* Effects of acupuncture treatment on daily life activities and quality of life. *Stroke* 1998;29:2100-8

BMA General Practitioners Committee. *Referrals to complementary therapists: guidance for GPs.* London: BMA GPC, 1999

Hadley CM. Complementary medicine and the general practitioner: a survey of general practitioners in the Wellington Area. *New Zealand Medical Journal* 1988;101:766-8

Halvorsen TB, Anda SS, Naess AB and Levang OW. Fatal cardiac tamponade after acupuncture through congenital sternal foramen. *The Lancet* 1995;345:1175

HL Hansard Vol. 610 29/2/00 WA63 (HL1144)

Harrington A (ed). *The Placebo Effect: an interdisciplinary exploration.* Cambridge, Mass.: Harvard University Press 1997

Hasegawa J, Noguchi N, Yamasaki J, Kotake H, Mashiba H, Sasaki S and Mori T. Delayed cardiac tamponade and haemothorax induced by an acupuncture needle. *Cardiology* 1991;78:58-63

Healthwork UK. *Standards and Qualifications: a consultation document for the complementary medicine sector.* London: Healthwork UK, May 1999

Healthwork UK. *National Occupational Standards for Homoeopathy.* IDeA publications: London, 2000.

Hopwood V. Acupuncture in physiotherapy. *Complementary Therapies in Medicine* 1993;1:100-4

Hu S, Stritzel R, Chandler A and Stern RM. P6 acupressure reduces symptoms of vection-induced motion sickness. *Aviation, Space and Environmental Medicine* 1995;66:631-4

Jadad AR, Moore RA, Carrol D, Jenkinson C, Reynolds DJM, Gavaghan DJ and McQuay HJ. Assessing the quality of reports of randomised clinical trials: is blinding necessary? *Controlled Clinical Trials* 1996;17:1-12

Jenkinson C and McGee H. *Health status measurement: a brief but critical introduction.* Oxford: Radcliffe Medical Press: 1998

Johansson K, Lindgren I, Widner H, Wiklund I and Johansson BB. Can sensory stimulation improve the functional outcome in stroke patients? *Neurology* 1993;43:2189-92

Kataoka HJ. Cardiac tamponade caused by penetration of an acupuncture needle into the right ventricle. *Journal of Thoracic and Cardiovascular Surgery* 1997;14:674-6

Knipschild P, Kleijnen J and ter Riet K. Belief in efficacy of alternative medicine among general practitioners in the Netherlands: Towards Acceptance and Integration. *Social Science and Medicine* 1990;31:625-6

Kohn M. *Complementary therapies in cancer care.* Abridged report of a study produced for Macmillan Cancer Relief: London, 1999

Lao L. Safety issues in acupuncture. *The Journal of Alternative and Complementary Medicine* 1996;2:27-31

Lautenschlaeger J. Akupunktur bei der Behandlung entzuendlich-rheumatischer Erkrankungen. *Zeitschrift fuer Rheumatologie* 1997;56:8-20

Lee A and Done ML. The use of nonpharmacologic techniques to prevent postoperative nausea and vomiting: a meta-analysis. *Anesthesia & Analgesia* 1999;88:1362-9

Lindall S. Is acupuncture for pain relief in general practice cost-effective? *Acupuncture in Medicine,* 1999;17:97-100

Linde K, Jobst K, Panton J. Acupuncture for chronic asthma (Cochrane Review). *The Cochrane Library, Issue 1, 2000.* Oxford: Update Software, 2000

Luff D and Thomas K. *Models of complementary therapy provision in primary care.* University of Sheffield: Medical Care Research Unit, 1999

MacLennan AH, Wilson DH and Taylor AW. Prevalence and cost of alternative medicine in Australia. *The Lancet* 1996;347:569-73

MacPherson H. Fatal and adverse events from acupuncture: allegation, evidence, and the implications. *The Journal of Alternative and Complementary Medicine* 1999;5:47-56

MacPherson H and Gould A. Grasping the nettle: a response to reports of adverse events from acupuncture. *The Journal of the Acupuncture Association of Chartered Physiotherapists* 1998;Autumn:8-14

Melchart D, Linde K, Fischer P, White A, Allais G, Vickers A and Berman B. Acupuncture for recurrent headaches: a systematic review of randomised controlled trials. *Cephalalgia* 1999;19:779-86

Mills SY. Safety awareness in complementary medicine. *Complementary Therapies in Medicine* 1996;4:48-51

Mills SY and Peacock W. *Professional organisation of complementary and alternative medicine in the United Kingdom.* Exeter University: The Centre for Complementary Health Studies, 1997

Mills SY and Budd S. *Professional organisation of complementary and alternative medicine in the United Kingdom.* Exeter University: The Centre for Complementary Health Studies, 2000

Morgan D, Glanville H, Mars S and Nathanson S. Education and training in complementary and alternative medicine: a postal survey of UK universities, medical schools and faculties of nurse education. *Complementary Therapies in Medicine* 1998;6:64-70

Murphy PA. Alternative therapies for nausea and vomiting of pregnancy. *Obstetrics and Gynaecology* 1998;91:149-55

Myers CP. Acupuncture in General Practice: Effect on drug expenditure. *Acupuncture in Medicine* 1991;9:71-2

National Health and Medical Research Council Study. *Acupuncture: a working party report.* Australian Government Publishing Service: Canberra, 1989

National Institutes of Health. *NIH Consensus Statement: Acupuncture.* 1997 Nov 3-5; 15:1-34

NHS Confederation. *Complementary medicine in the NHS: managing the issues.* Research Paper Number 4. Birmingham: The NHS Confederation, 1997

NHS Executive. *R&D in primary care: National working group report.* London: HMSO, November 1997

NHS Executive. *Developing primary care groups;* HSC 1998/139, London: NHSE, August 1998

Nieda S, Abe T, Kuribayashi R, Sato M and Abe S. Case of cardiac injury resulting from acupuncture. *Japanese Journal of Thoracic Surgery* 1973;26:881-3

Norheim AJ. Adverse effects of acupuncture: a study of the literature for the years 1981-1994. *The Journal of Alternative and Complementary Medicine* 1996;2:291-7

Norheim AJ and Fønnebø V. Adverse effects are more than occasional case reports: results from questionnaires among 1135 randomly selected doctors, and 197 acupuncturists. *Complementary Therapies in Medicine* 1996;4:8-13

Park J, White AR and Ernst E. Efficacy of acupuncture as a treatment for tinnitus: a systematic review. *Archives of Otolaryngology – Head and Neck Surgery;* in press

Perkin M, Pearcy R and Fraser J. A comparison of the attitudes shown by general practitioners, hospital doctors and medical students towards alternative medicine. *Journal of the Royal Society of Medicine* 1994;87:523-5

Pierfitte C, Begaud B, Lagnaoui R and Moore ND. Is reporting rate a good predictor of risks associated with drugs? *British Journal of Clinical Pharmacology* 1999;47:329-31

Pierik MG. Fatal staphylococcal septicemia following acupuncture: Report of two cases. *Rhode Island Medical Journal* 1982;65.251-3

Peuker ET and Filler TJ. The need for practical courses in anatomy for acupuncturists. *FACT* 1997;4:194

Rajanna P. Hypotension following stimulation of acupuncture point fengchi (GB 20). *Journal of the Royal College of General Practitioners* 1983;303:606-7

Rampes H. Adverse reactions to acupuncture. In: J Filshie, A White (eds) *Medical Acupuncture: A Western Scientific Approach.* Edinburgh: Churchill Livingstone, 1998

Rampes H and James R. Complications of acupuncture. *Acupuncture in Medicine* 1995;13:26-33

Rampes H and Peuker E. Adverse effects of acupuncture. In E Ernst and A White (eds) *Acupuncture: A scientific appraisal.* Oxford: Butterworth-Heinemann, 1999

Redfearn T. Oh, what a surprise! *Acupuncture in Medicine* 1991;9:2-3

Reilly D. Young doctors' views on alternative medicine. *British Medical Journal* 1983;87:337-9

Royal College of Physicians. *Science-based complementary medicine.* London: RCP, 1998

Royal London Homoeopathic Hospital. (2nd ed) *The evidence base of complementary medicine.* London: RLHH NHS Trust, 1999.

Royal London Homoeopathic Hospital. *The evidence base of complementary medicine.* London: RLHH NHS Trust, 1997

Royal Society. *Complementary and alternative medicine: response to the House of Lords inquiry into complementary and alternative medicine.* London: Royal Society, December 1999

Samuel O. Fundholding practices get preference. *British Medical Journal* 1992;305:1497

Schiff AF. A fatality due to acupuncture. *Medical Times (London)* 1965;93:630-1

Scottish Office Department of Health. *Complementary medicine and the National Health Service: an examination of acupuncture, homoeopathy, chiropractic and osteopathy.* London: HMSO, 1996

Shifrin K. Setting standards for acupuncture training – a model for complementary medicine. *Complementary Therapies in Medicine* 1995;3:13-5

Streitberger K and Kleinhenz J. Introducing a placebo needle into acupuncture research. *The Lancet* 1998;352:364-5

Tanii T, Kono T, Katoh J, Mizuno N, Fukuda M and Hamada T. A case of prurigo pigmentosa considered to be contact allergy to chromium in an acupuncture needle. *Acta Dermato-Venereologica* 1991;71:66-7

Thomas KJ, Fall M, Parry G, and Nicholl J. *National Survey of Access to Complementary Health Care via General Practice. DoH Report.* Sheffield: Medical Care Research Unit, 1995

Thomas K J and Fitter MJ. Evaluating complementary therapies for use in the National Health Service: 'Horses for courses'. Part 2: Alternative research strategies. *Complementary Therapies in Medicine* 1997;5:94-8

Thomas K J, Fitter M, Brazier J, MacPherson H, Campbell M, Nicholl J P and Roman M. Longer term clinical and economic benefits of offering acupuncture to patients with chronic low back pain assessed as suitable for primary care management. *Complementary Therapies in Medicine* 1999;7:91-100

Thomas KJ, Nicholl JP and Coleman P. Use and expenditure on complementary medicine in England – a population-based survey. *Complementary Therapies in Medicine* 2000; in press

Tramer MR, Moore RA, Reynolds DJ, McQuay HJ. Quantitative estimation of rare adverse events which follow a biological progression: a new model applied to chronic NSAID use. *Pain* 2000;85:169-82

Tuke J. Complication of acupuncture. *British Medical Journal* 1979;2:1076

Umlauf R. Analysis of the main results of the activity of the acupuncture department of faculty hospital. *Acupuncture in Medicine* 1988;5:16-18

van Haselen RA. The cost-effectiveness of complementary medicine: the current state of play. *The CompMed Supplement* 1999;1

van Haselen R and Fisher P. Attitudes to evidence on complementary medicine: the perspective of British healthcare purchasers. *Complementary Therapies in Medicine* 1999;7:125-98

van Tulder MW, Cherkin DC, Berman B, Lao L and Koes BW. The effectiveness of acupuncture in the management of acute and chronic low back pain. *Spine* 1999;24:1113-23

Venning P, Durie A, Roland M, Roberts C and Leese B. Randomised controlled trial comparing cost-effectiveness of general practitioners and nurse practitioners in primary care. *British Medical Journal* 2000;320:1048-53

Verhoef MJ and Sutherland LR. Alternative medicine and general practitioners: opinions and behaviour. *Canadian Family Physician* 1995;41:1005-11

Verma SK and Khamesra R. Recurrent fainting – an unusual reaction to acupuncture. *Journal of the Association of Physicians of India* 1989;37:600

Vickers AJ. Can acupuncture have specific effects on health? A systematic review of acupuncture antiemesis trials. *Journal of the Royal Society of Medicine* 1996;89:303-11

Visser D and Peters L. Alternative medicine and general practitioners in the Netherlands: Towards acceptance and integration. *Family Practice* 1990;7:227-32

Vittecoq D, Mettetal JF, Rouzioux C, Bach JF and Bouchon JP. Acute HIV infection after acupuncture treatments. *New England Journal of Medicine* 1989a;320:250-1

Vittecoq D, Mettetal JF, Rouzioux C, Bach JF and Bouchon JP. Unusual modes of HIV transmission. *New England Journal of Medicine* 1989b;321:1477

West Yorkshire Health Authority. *Guidelines for Employment of Complementary Therapists in the NHS* 1995/6. West Yorkshire Health Authority, September 1995

Wharton R and Lewith G. Complementary Medicine and the General Practitioner. *British Medical Journal* 1986;292:1498-1500

White A, Hayhoe S and Ernst E. Survey of adverse events following acupuncture. *Acupuncture in Medicine* 1997;15:67-70

White A, Rampes H and Ernst E. Acupuncture for smoking cessation. In: *The Cochrane Library Issue 4,* 1999. Oxford: Update Software, 1999

White A, Resch K-L and Ernst E. Methods of economic evaluation in complementary medicine. *Forschende Komplementärmedizin* 1996;3:196-203

White A, Resch K-L and Ernst E. Complementary medicine: use and attitudes among GPs. *Family Practice* 1997;14:302-6

White AR and Ernst E. A systematic review of randomised controlled trials of acupuncture for neck pain. *British Journal of Rheumatology* 1999;38:143-7

White AR and Ernst E. Economic analysis of complementary medicine: a systematic review. *Complementary Therapies in Medicine* 2000; 8:111-8

World Health Organisation. *Guidelines on Basic Training and Safety in Acupuncture,* Geneva: WHO, 1999

Worth C. Why and how the NHS is going complementary. *The Therapist,* 1995;Spring:9-12

Zollman C and Vickers A. ABC of Complementary medicine: Complementary medicine in conventional practice. *British Medical Journal* 1999;319:901-4

Index

123

DETROIT PUBLIC LIBRARY
BUSINESS, SCIENCE
AND TECHNOLOGY